Agile Actors on Complex Terrains

This book assesses the value and relevance of the literature on complex systems to policy-making, contributing to both social theory and policy analysis. For this purpose it develops two key ideas: agile action and transformative realism. The book takes some major themes from complexity science, presents them in a clear and accessible manner and applies them to core problems in sociological theory and policy analysis. Combining complexity science with perspectives from institutionalism and political economy, this book is the first to integrate these fields conceptually, methodologically and in terms of the implications for policy analysis and practice.

Room shows how the models and methods of social and complexity science can be jointly deployed and applied to empirical areas of public policy. He demonstrates how complexity science can provide insight into the nonlinear dynamics of the social world, but why these need to be understood by reference to the unequal distribution of power and advantage. Among the sociological debates with which the book engages are those concerned with causation and explanation, rational action and positional competition, and the place of evolutionary concepts in accounts of social change. Among the policy debates are those concerned with evidence and policy, the dynamics of inequality, and libertarian paternalism.

The book will appeal to final year undergraduates and postgraduate students in social sciences; scholars in social and policy studies broadly defined; policy-makers who want to go beyond conventional discussions of evidence-based policy-making and cross-national lesson-drawing, and consider how to approach complex and turbulent policy terrains; and a wider range of scholars in other disciplines where complexity science is already well developed.

Graham Room is Professor of European Social Policy at the University of Bath, UK.

Complexity in Social Science

This interdisciplinary series encourages social scientists to embrace a complex systems approach to studying the social world. A complexity approach to the social world has expanded across the disciplines since its emergence in the mid- to-late 1990s, and this can only continue as disciplines continue to change, data continue to diversify, and governance and responses to global social issues continue to challenge all involved. Covering a broad range of topics from big data and time, globalisation and health, cities and inequality, and methodological applications, to more theoretical or philosophical approaches, this series responds to these challenges of complexity in the social sciences – with an emphasis on critical dialogue around, and application of these ideas in, a variety of social arenas as well as social policy.

The series will publish research monographs and edited collections between 60,000–90,000 words that include a range of philosophical, methodological and disciplinary approaches, which enrich and develop the field of social complexity and push it forward in new directions.

David Byrne is Emeritus Professor at the School of Applied Social Sciences, Durham University, UK.

Brian Castellani is Professor in Sociology and Head of the Complexity in Health and Infrastructure Group, Kent State University, USA. He is also Adjunct Professor of Psychiatry, Northeastern Ohio Medical University.

Emma Uprichard is Associate Professor and Deputy Director at the Centre for Interdisciplinary Methodologies, University of Warwick, UK. She is also Co-Director of the Nuffield, ESRC, HEFCE funded Warwick Q-Step Centre.

Books:

Agile Actors on Complex Terrains
Transformative realism and public policy
Graham Room

Agile Actors on Complex Terrains

Transformative realism and public policy

Graham Room

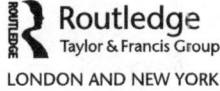
LONDON AND NEW YORK

First published 2016
by Routledge
2 Park Square, Milton Park, Abingdon, Oxon OX14 4RN

and by Routledge
711 Third Avenue, New York, NY 10017

Routledge is an imprint of the Taylor & Francis Group, an informa business

© 2016 Graham Room

The right of Graham Room to be identified as author of this work has been asserted by him in accordance with sections 77 and 78 of the Copyright, Designs and Patents Act 1988.

All rights reserved. No part of this book may be reprinted or reproduced or utilised in any form or by any electronic, mechanical, or other means, now known or hereafter invented, including photocopying and recording, or in any information storage or retrieval system, without permission in writing from the publishers.

Trademark notice: Product or corporate names may be trademarks or registered trademarks, and are used only for identification and explanation without intent to infringe.

British Library Cataloguing in Publication Data
A catalogue record for this book is available from the British Library

Library of Congress Cataloging in Publication Data
Names: Room, Graham, author.
Title: Agile actors on complex terrains : transformative realism and public
 policy / Graham Room.
Description: Abingdon, Oxon ; New York, NY : Routledge, 2017. | Series:
 Complexity in social science
Identifiers: LCCN 2016006770| ISBN 9781138959217 (hardback) |
 ISBN 9781315660769 (e-book)
Subjects: LCSH: Sociology—Philosophy. | Social sciences—Philosophy. |
 Complexity (Philosophy)
Classification: LCC HM585 .R66 2017 | DDC 301.01—dc23
LC record available at http://lccn.loc.gov/2016006770

ISBN: 978-1-138-95921-7 (hbk)
ISBN: 978-1-315-66076-9 (ebk)

Typeset in Times New Roman
by Swales & Willis Ltd, Exeter, Devon, UK

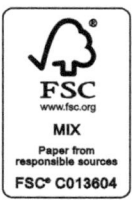

Printed and bound by CPI Group (UK) Ltd, Croydon, CR0 4YY

For Z
In memoriam

Contents

List of illustrations ix
Series editors' preface x
Acknowledgements xiv

Introduction 1

PART I
Transformative realism 7

1 Complexity and the social sciences 9
2 Evolution and the arts of civilisation 31
3 Contingent development and explanation
  (with Graham K. Brown) 50

PART II
Agile actors 75

4 Rationality, rationales and agile action 77
5 Positional advantage: a three-dimensional analysis 94
6 Navigating complex environments 110

PART III
Public policy 125

7 Evidence for agile policy-makers 127
8 Nudge or nuzzle? Improving decisions about active citizenship 146

9 Unequal rewards and the super-rich   164
   Conclusion   189

   Index   197

Illustrations

Figures

1.1	Svalbard	10
2.1	Fitness landscapes	38
3.1	The General Linear Model	51
3.2	Darwin's Tree of Life	56
3.3	The Contingent Historical Model	58
3.4	Creative destruction	60
3.5	Runaway loops	63
3.6	Jain and Krishna's autocatalytic sets	65
5.1	Fitness landscapes	103
7.1	The basic design of a Randomised Controlled Trial	129
7.2	Policy intervention as additive impact	130
7.3	Policy intervention as contingent diversification	132
7.4	Darwin's Tree of Life	133
7.5	Policy intervention as transformative synergy	135
7.6	Choosing a paradigm	136
9.1	Success as cumulative contingency: law firms	172

Table

7.1	Protocols for evidence	138

Series editors' preface

Graham Room is no stranger to the complexity sciences or their application to public policy. As Professor of European Social Policy, University of Bath, his involvement in this new interdisciplinary field began back in 2008, when he was awarded a two-year UK Research Fellowship from the ESRC (Economic and Social Research Council). The purpose of the grant was to explore the complexities of conceptualising and measuring dynamic change in social policy. Since then he has published a series of key articles, as well as his 2011 book, *Complexity, Institutions and Public Policy: Agile Decision-Making in a Turbulent World*.

Room admittedly turned to the complexity sciences in 2008 out of scholarly frustration. For him, while the outcomes-based, data-driven dynamics of social policy had grown more complex over the last few decades – particularly in terms of modelling turbulent social and economic change – the corresponding linear social science used to model these changes has woefully lagged behind, creating not only a major gap in understanding, but also the implementation of limited or, even worse, damaging public policy, particularly (as we have seen over the last ten years) in such areas as the international management of the global economic and political sectors, as in the case of the European Union and the Eurozone. By contrast, the complexity sciences offered Room (and those of similar mind) a new way of thinking about modelling social change, grounded in the epistemological assumption that social science (and its application to social policy) is best done from a complex systems perspective.

However, while the complexity sciences promise scholars like Room much in return for their hard work, it is not the case that all the concepts or methods or approaches from this thoroughgoing interdisciplinary field are scientifically equivalent; and it is not the case that all are equally equipped for modelling and implementing social policy – which brings us to the heart of our *Routledge Series on Complexity in Social Science* and to the heart of Room's book.

Like all authors in our series, Room has spent considerable time exploring the far-reaching complexity sciences, but not simply for the purposes of naively applying these ideas without thought. Instead, he has worked his way through the field (in deeply critical and often highly novel ways) to cull from it the intellectual concepts and techniques most useful to his particular area of social scientific inquiry, as well as (in many cases) social inquiry in general; which is why a book like Room's has such a wide intellectual appeal.

For example, effectively conceptualising and measuring dynamic change is not a problem limited to Room's concerns with social policy; instead, it is a problem of social science in general today – particularly given the challenges of big data and their related issues of time, evolution and dynamics! As such, taking the time to explore the hard-won insights of a scholar like Room (as well as the other writers in our series) can spark insights into other domains of inquiry, whether one is a complexity scientist or not. In fact, we hope that such a critical reading may even lead some readers, through their own dialogue with the series, to eventually publish in it; which takes us back to Room's book.

Room's *Agile Actors on Complex Terrains: Transformative Realism and Public Policy* picks up where his 2011 book (noted above) left off: further grounding policy studies in his novel (and, we must acknowledge, brilliant) integration of three intersecting fields of inquiry: complex systems theory, political economy, and institutionalism. Drawing upon these three fields, the crux of Room's argument is based on two key ideas, around which he develops a series of novel and highly useful insights, concepts and policy-based recommendations. The first is *complex terrains*; and the second is *agile action on this complex terrain*.

Room's concept of *complex terrains*, at least initially, draws heavily upon complex systems theory. For Room, we live, today, in a high-dynamic, relatively turbulent, nonlinear, far-from-equilibrium, globally interdependent world. At the macroscopic level, the world tends to give the impression of being low dynamic; particularly as experienced by those living in affluent western societies; or by those living in poverty trap countries impervious to external improvement or change. Such macroscopic stabilities are nonetheless contingent upon a continuous process of microscopic and mesoscopic flows, variations, perturbations and radical transformation; which, as the last decade of global events has demonstrated, can suddenly lead to significant macroscopic change. Easy examples are the United States banking scandal and its corresponding global financial crisis; the Arab Spring and the destabilisation of Afghanistan; the political collapse of Syria and the outmigration of refugees into Europe; the halting Chinese market and its ownership of foreign debt; Russia's invasion of the Ukraine and its threat to European stability; and the significant volatility of the European Union and Eurozone due to the national debt of countries such as Italy and Greece.

To make sense of this world, and the development of effective policy to manage it, one needs something slightly more sophisticated than convention – argues Room – with its reductionist linear modelling, equilibrium-based economics, rational action/choice theory, and its all-too-often local bias toward privileged self-interest or country. One needs, instead, a *complex systems view of the world*, which helps us understand the dynamic feedback loops between multifaceted and multilevel policy and practice.

But that is not all, Room argues. One also needs the insights of institutionalism and political economy. For Room, while the complexity sciences offer a powerful lens for viewing and modelling the complex, high-dynamic terrain in which public policy is situated, this lens tends toward the microscopic; that is, it over-emphasises the role of agent-based actions and the behavioural economics of interacting people and groups. As a result, the complexity sciences have insufficiently developed a corresponding framework for making sense of the larger co-present and co-determining organisational patterns in which multi-agent behaviour is situated, as in the case of macroscopic political and institutional power or economic conflict and group privilege.

In short, contra complexity science and the psychologically oriented conventions of current policy study, it is insufficient to view policy-making as little more than a Schelling-like model of microscopic agents, as they evolve, across time and space, into complex networks of interaction, all taking place on some complex two-dimensional simulated grid. Needed, as well, is an understanding of the larger institutional arrangements in which these microscopic, policy-based interactions take place, as well as the organisational patterns of political economy, as they take the form of various historically contingent mesoscopic and macroscopic structures – all of which leads to Room's second key idea, *agile action on complex terrain*.

For Room, *agile action on complex terrain* is about developing a more nuanced understanding of how social actors and social policy move through and within the complex topography of various communities, countries or regions, as situated within globalised society. In strong contrast to the rationalist or behaviourist models that currently dominate the field, Room shows us a multilevel landscape of dynamic uncertainty, with flexible actors and institutions involved in partial-knowledge-based negotiations; where some groups or organisations, given various institutional arrangements, are far more privileged in their position and power and understanding and access to resources than others; all of which pushes policy-making toward a more 'complex systems' understanding of economic and political behaviour and outcomes grounded in (his words) a 'social distribution of uncertainty', as well as 'the purposive probing of agile actors and their struggles for positional advantage'. In other words, Room is clear: the interdependent complexities of power and position and structure are central to any understanding of public policy, no matter how complex the model. And, if there is any hope for civilised order or economic and social well-being for all, it is grounded in such an understanding of the world and its management. The rest is folly.

From here, Room uses his idea of *complex terrains* and *agile actions* to develop an equally impressive list of related concepts and insights, all provocative and compelling in their own right. Here are a few examples: (1) given the turbulence involved in social change, the field of policy studies should be an *evolutionary complex systems science*; (2) because of the role that time and contingency play in social dynamics, we would be better served to adopt a *contingent historical model of social change*; (3) any understanding of policy implementation requires an understanding of how *agile actors 'read', in 'real time', the policies they enact*; and (4) while *nudge-based policy*, which is heavily psychological in focus, tends to see citizens as implementers of existing policy (think, for example of behavioural economics and discounting theory), *nuzzle-based policy*, grounded in political economy, sees citizens as *co-creators of public policy*, seeking to 'nuzzle' their talents and abilities and concerns into the interdependent networks of economic and political influence and security and stability in which they live.

There is much more in Room's book, but we will stop there, passing the front-stage lectern to him instead. Still, as we hope this brief introduction to Room suggests – and, in turn, we hope this series will inspire – there is much to be gained from a critical dialogue with the complexity sciences and, more specifically, complex systems theory, as the world in which we currently live, along with the massive global problems we presently face, appear far too scientifically demanding otherwise. In fact, to turn a phrase by Steven Hawking, the complexity sciences, if developed correctly, could become the best of social inquiry as practised in the twenty-first century.

Dave Byrne, Brian Castellani and Emma Uprichard
Complexity in Social Science series editors

Acknowledgements

The ideas here were developed during a sabbatical year spent in part at Policy Horizons Canada in Ottawa, the Institute for Governance and Policy Studies, Victoria University, Wellington, and Korea University, Seoul. I am grateful to colleagues at all of these institutions for comments on earlier versions of various chapters.

Many colleagues at my own university have given generously of their time to read these ideas in draft. I mention in particular Graham K. Brown (now at the University of Western Australia), who collaborated in the writing of Chapter 3; Jean Boulton, whose own book *Embracing Complexity* was published in 2015 by Oxford University Press; and James Copestake, whose work applies complexity ideas to a wide range of development contexts. Hester Kan read most of the chapters in their final version and made many useful suggestions for improvement.

The book builds in part on a programme of work supported by the Economic and Social Research Council (Award RES-063-27-0130) and my book *Complexity, Institutions and Public Policy: Agile Decision-Making in a Turbulent World*, Cheltenham: Edward Elgar (2011).

A version of the material in Chapter 2 previously appeared in the journal *Policy and Politics*; Chapter 7 in *Evidence and Policy*; and Chapter 8 in *Policy Studies*. I am grateful to the editors and publishers in each case for permission to draw here on those earlier versions.

I am grateful to Wiley publishers for permission to reproduce, as Figure 3.6, part of a diagram from S. Bornholdt and H.G. Schuster (eds), *Handbook of Graphs and Networks*, Weinheim: Wiley-VCH, pp. 355–95.

All web pages cited were operational when this manuscript was submitted to the publisher.

Department of Social and Policy Sciences
University of Bath
http://www.bath.ac.uk/sps/staff/graham-room/

Introduction

This book is concerned with public policy and the social science on which it draws.

How are we to visualise the policy world? One metaphor is the putting green. On this uniform terrain, the golfer can hit the ball in a simple application of Newton's laws of motion. True, there may be a gentle slope and the golfer may misjudge the degree of friction that the well-manicured grass affords: but slight adjustments when striking the ball will readily compensate for these. Policy-makers on such terrains, equipped with reliable evidence of the effectiveness of different interventions, can deploy whichever they deem most appropriate, with some confidence as to the results.

The real world of policy-making may, however, be less like a putting green than a game of crazy golf, with hills, valleys and obstacles making for a landscape that is far from uniform. Worse still, the golfer may discover that the game is being played on a 'bouncy castle' of the sort that is now commonplace in children's playgrounds. Now, as the ball is struck and proceeds on its course, its weight modifies the topology of the golf course itself. With multiple players, all active on the same terrain, rational policy-making may seem quite impossible.

This world of valleys, hills and malleable topographies involves feedback loops, so that as the various actors pursue their own objectives, they change the ground which other actors then face. This turbulence has become only too apparent in recent years, with the international financial and economic crisis spilling over to affect all areas of public policy. Government leaders warn that conventional methods of policy intervention no longer seem to work. New models of a dynamically interconnected world are needed, if they are to anticipate, steer and control this turbulence.

Of course, there is much that remains stable: otherwise we would hardly be able to live our everyday lives. Policy terrains are interconnected, but only up to a point. Social institutions – the school, the workplace, the associations within the local community – enforce their respective rules and give some order to our lives. Nevertheless, it is easy to take their order for granted; to assume that this order is unchanging; and not to notice the small changes that are continuously under way. It is easy to be blind to the fragility and contingent nature of these institutions, and to the 'weak signals' of imminent 'tipping points' that may herald their dramatic transformation. It is also easy to focus on the stability that may be evident at home, while overlooking developments elsewhere. The long and oft-celebrated period of stability enjoyed by Victorian England was accompanied by immense disruption to the indigenous peoples of her expanding world empire.

This book assesses the value and relevance to policy-making of the literature on complex systems. This recognises the *non-linear, path-dependent* and often *counter-intuitive* dynamics of the policy world. It also recognises that no policy is launched onto a greenfield site: it is an intervention in a tangled web of institutions that have developed incrementally over extended periods of time and through a succession of political struggles. These give each policy context its own specificity. Therefore, while complexity analysis can play a central and essential role in the analysis of policy dynamics, it must be combined with an appreciation of institutions and political economy.

This book contributes to both social theory and policy analysis. For this purpose it develops two key ideas: *agile action* and *transformative realism*. Here we introduce each of these notions and draw some implications for public policy analysis.

Agile action

If we need to rethink our view of policy terrains, the same goes for our view of the social actors who move on those terrains. Rational action theories remain dominant across much of social science, with social actors assessing the menu of choices available to them in terms of their costs, benefits and consequences. There is, however, increasing recognition of the bounds to such rationality, because of the partial information that actors have at their disposal and their limited ability to assess risk. This was evident, for example, in the 2008 financial crisis, when the 'rationality' of the financiers produced risky behaviours that almost led to systemic collapse.

Meanwhile, recent years have seen growing interest – especially on the part of economists – in behaviourist perspectives. These, to some degree, abandon orthodox models of rational economic behaviour, especially as far as 'ordinary' people are concerned, instead pointing to the biases and blunders that they display in many of their decisions. These behaviourist perspectives have increased the attention given in policy debate not only to the contribution of psychologists but also that of neuroscientists, claiming to measure well-being in a far more rigorous manner than social scientists could ever offer.

This book will challenge many of these perspectives. It will offer instead an account in terms of *agile actors*. This depicts social actors as probing the complex and turbulent landscapes on which they find themselves, but only if they can do so from the vantage point of some stable and settled ground. In contrast to rational action theories, it sees social actors not as menu-takers but as menu-shapers, reworking and contesting the social and economic world in which they find themselves. In contrast to behaviourist perspectives, it understands any biases and blunders by reference to the settled ground from which social actors draw their routines and practices: a ground which must be understood in terms not of psychology but of sociology and political economy. The result is a perspective on social action that sharply distances itself from the abstract individualism of much contemporary writing.

We give a central place to uncertainty and to the efforts by agile actors to offload its costs onto others. The social distribution of uncertainty – and of the turbulence to which we have referred – therefore moves centre-stage. But of course, this is a struggle played on unequal terms. Those already at a positional disadvantage are likely to carry a disproportionate share. They may end up with hardly any stable and settled ground from which to shape their world: and with little option, therefore, but to hunker down and cling to a precarious existence.

Transformative realism

How are we to explain social regularities and patterns? The 'realist' tradition in the philosophy of science gives pride of place to the generative processes or mechanisms which produce such phenomena and the various contingencies to which they are subject.

Agile social actors probe the complex and turbulent landscapes on which they find themselves. They experiment and they learn. They attempt to discover dynamic synergies on the landscapes of their world, which they can mobilise to their own advantage. In analysing the transformations they produce, the focus is not, therefore, on the individual actor or policy intervention, but on the dynamic interactions that develop and the blockages that they face, all located within the institutional and political struggles which have shaped the society in question. We refer to this perspective as *transformative realism*, and around this we develop our methodological position.

The complexity literature – drawing heavily upon the natural and informational sciences – offers a wide range of models for understanding the patterns of 'self-organisation' and 'emergence' in complex systems. This book makes use of those models – but always insisting that in the social sciences those emerging patterns must be understood by reference to the purposive probing of agile actors and their struggles for positional advantage.

Darwin (1859) often insists: '*Natura non facit saltum*' (nature makes no leaps). Kauffman (1993), one of the classic writers on complex systems, also highlights the risks attached to 'long jumps' on complex terrains. Nevertheless, agile social actors know that under some conditions small actions may – through the dynamic synergies they generate – lead to disproportionate effects. Smart long jumps, exploiting these transformative synergies, may therefore be possible. Moreover, the rewards may be great, especially if the risks and costs of change can be deflected onto others. This underlines, however, that transformation for one person may mean disruption, turbulence and uncertainty for another.

Much of the complexity literature is concerned with a multitude of individual agents aware only of their immediate local situations. From these local interactions, amazing macro-formations can emerge. This must not, however, lead us to overlook the ways that human actors can draw on their organised collective imagination and intelligence, in pursuit of smart long jumps and the transformations they promise.

Public policy

Complex dynamics can produce a tangled knot of institutions and policy interventions, with path dependencies and lock-ins which are hard to escape, and trade-offs which allow of no easy resolution. These are sometimes described as 'wicked' problems.

Policy interventions launched with insufficient thought as to their interactions with the wider policy ecosystem are unlikely to be sufficient to the task. In contrast, taking those interactions into account may enable the transformative long jumps to which we have just referred. This is why Hirschman, for example, faced with the challenge of under-development, argues for policy interventions that can produce a succession of 'imbalances, tensions, disproportions and disequilibria', chosen so as to stimulate investment and entrepreneurship across the society at large. This involves government watching how the wider economy organises itself around the interventions in question, with a view to nurturing the dynamic synergies that then unfold. This involves a continuing 'dance' between the self-organisation that may 'emerge' and the efforts of policy-makers – and indeed other strategic actors – to impose organisation and direction of their own.

This is a rather different vision from that of Hayek and his followers. For Hayek (1948), central planning and government direction contradict accounts of the economy as a complex system. The central planner can never bring together all the information that such an economy entails: it is much better to leave the myriad interacting agents to self-organise. Free markets, if left to themselves, will deliver efficiency and wealth, distributed to the different factors of production according to their respective contributions. Government should, therefore, limit itself to promoting the creativity of citizens and securing the good order of the market.

Keynes (1936) doubted this. He questioned whether, under conditions of uncertainty, a modern economy could ever self-organise at full employment of national resources and economic capacity, without the active intervention of the State. This Keynesian perspective has been given added salience by the turbulence that followed the recent economic crisis. Moreover, as warned by Polanyi (1944), if markets are left to 'self-organise', this seems to produce social consequences, in terms of social inequality and insecurity, that undermine social consent and threaten a backlash against the very market institutions on which prosperity depends. In any case, the market as envisaged by Hayek – with myriad autonomous decision-makers – is hardly the market of the modern world, dominated as it is by large corporations, the real 'central planners' of the global economy.

The societies of today are characterised by great inequalities of power and advantage. If public policy analysis is to take inspiration from the complexity literature, it must consider critically the terms on which different groups of social actors are involved in the policy 'dance': whether pursuing their respective purposes, probing and transforming the terrains across which they live their lives, or limited to a marginal and precarious existence. It is from this vantage point that we will tackle some of the public policy issues of today.

The book is organised into three main parts: concerned, respectively, with transformative realism, agile action and public policy. The chapters in each of these three parts elaborate and develop the three sections of this Introduction. There is a developing argument through the book: nevertheless, the chapters are sufficiently free-standing that they can also be read individually.

Less time is spent than in my previous book (Room, 2011) on exposition of the various strands of complexity writing: the reader who wants a more extensive introduction should consult that earlier volume. Attention instead focuses on some of the major methodological and conceptual debates in social science to which the complexity literature is relevant and on the forms of public policy analysis that flow from these. What unites the two books is a belief that model-building and empirical analysis must go hand in hand: and that any complexity perspective applied to the social world must be grounded in the institutional analysis and political economy of the societies in question.

References

Darwin, C. (1859), *The Origin of Species,* London: Wordsworth (reprinted 1998)
Hayek, F. (1948), *Individualism and Economic Order,* Chicago: Chicago University Press
Kauffman, S.A. (1993), *The Origins of Order: Self-Organisation and Selection in Evolution,* Oxford: Oxford University Press
Keynes, J.M. (1936), *The General Theory of Employment, Interest and Money,* London: Macmillan
Polanyi, K. (1944), *The Great Transformation,* New York: Rinehart
Room, G. (2011), *Complexity, Institutions and Public Policy: Agile Decision-Making in a Turbulent World,* Cheltenham: Edward Elgar

Part I
Transformative realism

1 Complexity and the social sciences

1.1 Introduction

Sociology has long been concerned with the relationship between social action and agency at the micro-level and social structure and order at the macro-level.

New insights into this relationship are offered by the literature on complex systems (Room, 2011a). A complex system involves elements that interact with each other but also with their larger environment. The complexity literature lays bare the conditions under which these micro-interactions can generate order or structure at the macro-level, even in the absence of any overarching system of control. This may explain the eagerness of social scientists, over the last decade, to apply these insights to the social world.[1]

The literature on complex systems springs largely from the natural and informational sciences. This chapter examines the distinctive contribution which the literature on complex systems may offer to the social sciences. Unsurprisingly, some of the same questions posed in earlier methodological disputes around the social and natural sciences reappear here.

The first step is to examine the dynamics of complex systems in relation to the natural and informational sciences. The second is to interrogate some of the major sociological debates on the emergence of macro-patterns from micro-interactions and to clarify in what respects the social world is different. Later sections of the chapter consider the implications for theory-building and method.

1.2 The emergence of order in complex systems

Complex systems, to repeat, involve elements that interact with each other, but also with their larger environment. These are, therefore, not closed but *open* systems, which encounter both positive and negative feedback from the larger environment in which they are embedded, and which they simultaneously reshape. Negative feedback tends to mean that the system stays the same: this is what is assumed in models of static equilibrium. Positive feedback means that any change will tend to be self-reinforcing, irreversible and path-dependent. These negative and positive feedbacks can involve the emergence of orderly patterns across the system and the larger environment in which it sits. This is what complexity writers refer to as 'self-organisation'.

10 *Transformative realism*

The micro-level interactions among the elements of such systems mean that the emerging patterns are in various degrees non-linear: they involve more than the simple aggregation of changes in the individual elements. These patterns can be quite counter-intuitive and their contours may change dramatically, if the interactions shift even in quite small ways. The complexity literature offers a variety of models for making sense of such non-linear processes and the dramatic alterations in dynamics that they can display: these have been powerfully and fruitfully applied across many different fields. Nevertheless, not everything interacts with everything else: there is much in the world that is stable and predictable and that linear models are well able to illuminate.

The literature on complex systems has captured the interest of a wide variety of social scientists. However, in order to assess this promise, we must first notice what is involved in its use within the natural and informational sciences. Only then can we assess its possible application, *mutatis mutandis*, to the social world, and the perils and benefits this may bring.

The following photograph (Figure 1.1) was taken in Svalbard. Here is a hillside whose upper reaches are continuously being turned into gravel by erosion. Gravity moves the gravel downwards, so that it piles up along the horizontal escarpments that run along lower reaches of the hillside.

In many places along these escarpments, the particles now begin to spill over, forming small fissures as they do so. Some fissures develop more quickly than others: it is these that 'capture' flows of material that might have escaped along

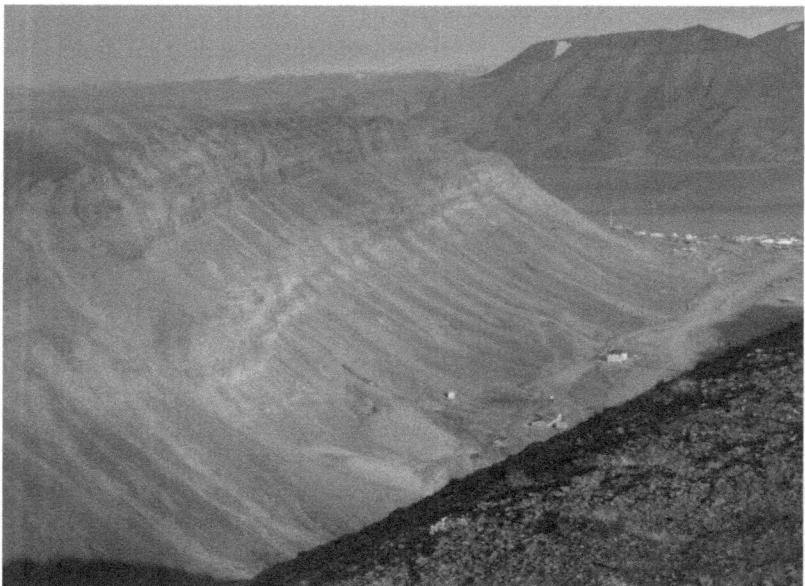

Figure 1.1 Svalbard

other routes and, in doing so, they become bigger still. This is a form of positive feedback. The result is a process of self-organisation in terms of these striations, distributed at regular intervals along the escarpment.

This self-organisation has come, we might say, at a price: the elimination of all those mini-fissures that began forming, but were then swamped and incorporated by their more developed neighbours, as they dragged in material from the larger hillside. In this way the process of self-organisation has 'simplified' the escarpment, as lots of mini-fissures were eliminated and a starker and more sharply defined topography 'emerged'.

The size of the intervals between fissures depends on such factors as the typical size of the gravel particles and their coefficients of friction. Change these and the interval would be different: indeed, the topography and dynamic development of the whole hillside might well change. In the language of complex systems, these variables are the 'control parameters' of such dynamics.

A second example taken from the physical world might be the development of our Solar System, as planets formed out of stellar dust (Stewart, 2003). The more massive the planets that form, the more they warp the space-time environment in which other celestial bodies find themselves, dragging those other bodies towards them, by what for shorthand we call 'gravity'. The concentration of matter thereby confers increasing structure on the space-time environment. These are self-reinforcing processes that warp ever-wider expanses of the universe. At the same time, the process hoovers up a host of minor bodies. This parallels the emergence of an orderly pattern of striations on the hills of Svalbard.

To conclude: These processes of dynamic change, within open and complex systems, involve self-organisation and the emergence of structure: at the same time, however, they also involve the obliteration and recycling of alternative bases of organisation.[2]

Biologists have been no less eager, *mutatis mutandis*, to apply the ideas behind complex systems to the living world. Living systems are, of course, physical systems and subject to the laws of physics. But they are more than that. Here we ask: in what sense do living systems encounter positive and negative feedback from the larger environment in which they are embedded, and which they simultaneously reshape? The answer is given in part by evolutionary science, concerned with the dynamic transformation of an ancient world (Crutchfield and Schuster, 2003). Here the driver is not gravity but what Darwin described as the 'struggle for existence', as a vast number of organisms compete desperately for food and mates. They also produce new generations of offspring: some of these exhibit variations which confer advantage in the struggle, within the particular environment in question. Here, as before, is a system whose elements are interacting more or less vigorously with each other and with the larger world.

Just as the downward flows of sand-like material on Svalbard's heights produce the regular striations described above, the selective environment of the 'struggle for existence' produces, over many generations, an ecosystem of species finely adjusted to their habitats. Flannery (1994) compares the evolutionary biology of the lands of Australasia. In New Zealand, birds came to dominate; in New Caledonia, reptiles; in Australia, marsupials. Across these different ecosystems, Flannery identifies equivalent niches for particular birds, reptiles and marsupials, respectively, the counterparts of the major species of placental mammals on the Eurasian landmass. These, he argues, are regularities set by the interdependence of evolutionary niches. This is what Kauffman (1993, 1995), one of the principal writers on evolutionary biology as a complex system, calls 'order for free'.

This process of selection also includes the dynamics of co-evolution. This involves positive dynamic synergies and feedback, for example between flowering plants and insects. These progressively come to dominate the ecosystems in which they are involved, limiting the scope for other species to thrive or even rendering them extinct. It is the latter that are the 'waste' of these self-organising dynamics, the alternative bases of organisation that are obliterated and recycled. Here again apparently small changes in such ecosystems – the disappearance for example of a particular species – can mean a dramatic shift in the system's dynamics. Even so, ecosystems can also display long periods of stability and resilience in face of fluctuations within their environment (Solé and Bascompte, 2006).[3]

From the natural world we turn finally to the application of the literature on complex systems to the study of human societies. Human societies involve living systems and living systems are made up of physical systems. They are, therefore, subject to the laws of both physics and evolutionary biology. But they are more than that.

Here are social actors interacting vigorously with each other and with the larger social world: they are the 'animating principles' of the social (Popper, 1994). Here also are social structures and patterns at the macro-level. How far can these be explained by reference to processes of emergence analogous to those we have described for the physical and biological worlds; and what are the limitations of such explanations?

This provides the agenda for the rest of this chapter. Nevertheless, in exploring these disciplinary affinities, we do well to take into account, more than has sometimes been done by those applying complexity ideas to the social world, the cautions developed through earlier methodological disputes around the social and natural sciences.

1.3 Social emergence and explanation

We need to look at how human actors and human societies encounter positive and negative feedback from the larger environment in which they are embedded, and which they simultaneously reshape. We must see how far forms of self-organisation emerge. And we must see in what ways this involves the obliteration and recycling of alternative bases of organisation. Such processes are well represented in Kuhn's account of how natural science itself develops, centred as this is on the emergence of new paradigms of scientific thought and practice – and their corollary, the disorganisation, obliteration and recycling of the orthodoxies they replace (Kuhn, 1970). Now, however, we widen our interest to social dynamics more generally.

In broad terms it is not difficult to see these basic elements of complex systems reflected in a variety of social science writing. Sociology, in particular, has long been concerned with the relationship between social action and agency at the micro-level and social structure and order at the macro-level. Thus, for example, Marx, Parsons and Giddens grapple with how to combine agency and social structure in a dynamic analysis that recognises their interdependence: and these questions maintain their relevance within contemporary debates.

How social science conceptualises 'macro' – and its relationship to the micro-level – is, however, not unproblematic. For orthodox economics, the macro-level is a marketplace of perfect information and perfect competition, driving the behaviour of micro-actors towards equilibrium. Such equilibrium thinking has long been the target of criticism by a wide range of heterodox economists (see, for example, Kaldor, 1985). Very different is the perspective of evolutionary economists such as Dopfer and Potts (2008), who approach the macro-level instead in terms of the co-evolutionary dynamics of the economy as a whole. This resonates closely with our earlier account of open systems.

In sociology, Dawe (1970) identified two main perspectives. He described, first, the 'sociology of order'. Here the macro-level is a fixed, exogenous and more or less coherent 'context', constraining the micro-behaviour of individual actors. Thus, for example, Durkheim portrayed the 'macro-level' as constituted by a variety of social forces, including the 'suicidogenic currents' that govern rates of suicide and give them their stability (Durkheim, 1897/1952). These currents can arise from various forms of breakdown in social cohesion, including those associated with rapid industrialisation and urbanisation. Dawe then contrasts the 'sociology of order' with the 'sociology of control'. This centres on the efforts of social actors to construct and reconstruct the social order in which they find themselves and to impose their meanings and purposes upon it. Here the macro-level is the outcome – at any particular moment – of the struggles for control and emancipation in which individual actors are involved. It may exhibit some degree of order but there is likely to be plenty of disorder also.

In what follows we focus on some of the more empirically focused attempts at a sociology that spans micro and macro, social action and social structure. All adopt a broadly Weberian approach to the explanation of social patterns and regularities: accepting Weber's dictum that such explanations must on the one hand be consistent with the statistical regularities at macro-level that empirical research adduces ('causal adequacy'), while also being true to the subjective meanings that the actors in question give to their actions ('adequacy at the level of meaning') (Weber, 1949).

We begin with perspectives that move from micro to macro by simple aggregation. We then turn to a variety of other sociological contributions which move beyond these limitations, and which consider in particular how:

14 *Transformative realism*

- micro-actions produce macro-changes which self-organise;
- social actors search purposefully for these transformative macro-dynamics;
- social actors draw on the macro-level so as to enhance their capacity to lever change.

In this way we flesh out a sociological perspective on emergence which resonates with the foregoing discussion of complex systems, but which also recognises the distinguishing features of the social world.

Micro and macro in a linear world

Goldthorpe (2007a, 2007b) places the link between micro and macro at the centre of his attention. The task of the sociologist is to establish what social regularities there are at a macro-level and to explain these by reference to the social actions that are taken by a multiplicity of individuals at the micro-level (Goldthorpe, 2007a: ch. 9).

He argues that if these myriad actions have a general tendency in a particular direction, albeit with fluctuations around this that are more or less random, we can expect that the aggregate of these actions will be in that same direction (Goldthorpe, 2007a: 128–9). The task of the sociologist is to detect this general tendency at the micro-level and to confirm the resulting aggregate pattern at the macro-level. In these circumstances the aggregation from micro to macro involves little more than simple addition.

Goldthorpe recognises that social actors are variously located within structures of hierarchical differentiation, involving unequal advantage and power (Goldthorpe and Bevan, 1977). In his studies of social mobility, he reckons that as a general tendency, they purposefully deploy their positions of advantage and power to secure and advance the opportunities of their offspring (Goldthorpe, 2007b: 9). It is hardly surprising then that the inequalities in the mobility chances of each generation remain rather stable, as Goldthorpe's empirical studies have robustly demonstrated. The relative chances enjoyed by offspring tend to reflect the advantages or disadvantages of their parents. By capturing this general tendency at the micro-level and aggregating to the macro-level, Goldthorpe abstracts from the micro-fluctuations and 'noise', and reckons to have thereby explained the stability in intergenerational mobility chances.

This approach may work well in many situations. Nevertheless, it may be insufficient to treat the macro-regularities that we observe in empirical data sets as the linear aggregation of myriad micro-choices. Social actors not only act, they also interact. This can set non-linear processes in motion, which may transform those macro-regularities in new directions. Certainly our discussion of complexity perspectives suggested that this was potentially important.

This is not all. Goldthorpe argues that purpose-rational action must be centre-stage in sociological explanation (see Chapter 4 for more detailed discussion). Here the social actor is confronted with a range of options, carrying particular costs, benefits and consequences. However, it is also rational for social actors to reshape the menu of options, where this is possible, so as to make them more attractive. Their leverage and scope for doing this will depend upon where they sit within the society's various structures of hierarchical differentiation, and the resources and connections these make available. This again means that linear aggregation of micro-choices will not suffice.

Micro-actions produce macro-changes which self-organise

Hedström (2005) builds on the legacy of Coleman (1990). Like Goldthorpe, he accepts that sociology must develop explanations of macro-level phenomena which articulate with social action at the micro-level. However, Hedström focuses on the micro-level interactions among actors and the macro-patterns to which these can give rise: patterns which are not, *pace* Goldthorpe, the simple aggregation of those individual actions and which may indeed take forms that are counter-intuitive. He uses formal mathematical modelling or, when faced with non-linear systems not tractable by formal mathematical methods, he turns to computational methods. Agent-based modelling is here his main tool, building on the work of such writers as Schelling and Holland.

Schelling (1978: ch. 4) is one of the classics of the complexity literature. His agents have different addresses on a grid or lattice. Schelling posits a 'tolerance schedule', a preference not to have within one's immediately adjacent neighbourhood more than a certain proportion of another race: the general racial composition of the city at large is, however, of no concern. Starting with an initially random distribution of households across the city, Schelling conducts repeated simulations, as households walk step-wise to an adjacent address, whenever their immediate neighbours exceed this racial threshold. He shows that even a rather mild level of racial antipathy – and concerned only with immediate neighbours – will quickly generate zones of racial segregation across the city.

Schelling's actors react to the racial composition of their immediate neighbourhood. As they do so however, their actions affect the composition of adjacent neighbourhoods, and the society as a whole moves progressively to a more segregated state. Any particular individual may find that, whatever the level of their own tolerance, the ethnic composition of their neighbourhood is increasingly likely to exceed that threshold, obliging them to move. Alternatively, even the most tolerant may find that their neighbourhood steadily loses all diversity. In this way the rate of segregation accelerates, through the processes of positive feedback to which we referred when introducing the literature on complex systems earlier in this chapter. This has been termed 'downward causation' (Campbell, 1974; Noble, 2006: ch. 4).

In Schelling's model, the tolerance level for residents of the city is the 'control parameter' of the dynamics that then unfold. Depending on the value that this takes, the city may see minimal movement, or the self-reinforcing processes of progressive segregation just discussed, or a chaotic flux. The city will, moreover, shift between these very different macro-dynamics at very narrowly defined 'tipping points' or 'bifurcations'. This is a common feature of such non-linear systems.[4]

16 *Transformative realism*

Just as Schelling demonstrates how the homogenous clustering of racial groups develops, Hedström (2005: ch. 6) develops agent-based models of young people in Stockholm, adjusting to the unemployment experience of their neighbours. He recognises that such models must be empirically grounded and calibrated. He checks how far the model produces clustering that approximates to the spatial maps of youth unemployment revealed by the Stockholm statistics. Hedström reckons that this provides an explanatory bridge between micro and macro: consistent with the macro-statistics but also 'adequate at the level of meaning'.

Unlike Schelling, Hedström discusses institutional contexts and the scope for individuals to re-weave them. He stresses that the structural configurations in which actors are embedded are fateful for the social outcomes that emerge; and that agents interact 'under conditions inherited from the past' (2005: 98–9). He also recognises that individuals may have a wide range of possible beliefs and desires informing their actions. Nevertheless, these insights hardly enter into his formal modelling.

Beyond Schelling and Hedström, there are many other agent-based computational models that explore such non-linear emergence: in other words, how micro-actions can produce macro-changes which self-organise (see, for example, the *Journal of Artificial Societies and Social Simulation*). However, they generally suffer from the same limitations as those we have just identified. Beyond this agent-based modelling, there are other models of 'emergence' and 'self-organisation' that spring from the natural sciences but have been applied to social phenomena (see, for example, Ball (2004) and Room (2011a)). We will return to some of these later in this chapter.

Social actors search purposefully for these transformative macro-dynamics

In Schelling, micro-actors pay no attention to the macro-structures that emerge: this takes place behind their backs, so to speak, or above their heads. However, in the real world, social actors have some inkling of these macro-processes. They probe purposefully and they try – depending on the resources and power at their disposal – to modify and reshape this 'downward causation' to their own ends. Instead of just being menu-takers, they are also in some degree menu-makers. They attempt to make their own history, albeit in circumstances not entirely of their own choosing. These efforts are, however, liable to be contested by others (Bronowski, 1981).

This purposeful search is central to Dawe's (1970) 'sociology of control': focused on social action that looks for positional advantage, emancipation and control of the contingencies of life, while offloading uncertainty and insecurity onto others. The order that emerges is then in some degree the deliberate – if also contested – result of these efforts; so too is the recycling and obliteration of alternative bases of organisation. This strategic agency and purposeful opportunism distinguish the social world from the dynamics of the natural world, from whose study the complexity literature has in considerable measure emerged.

Within the social science literature, there are plenty of examples of just such a perspective. Crouch (2005) examines purposeful opportunism and strategic agency in relation to the array of institutions with which we are each confronted. He castigates rational action theory for its assumption of 'institution-takers' rather than 'institution-makers'. In real life, 'aggressively maximising entrepreneurial actors must be expected to challenge all conventions and rules that shape their opportunities and environment' (p. 68). Rational action theory denies such entrepreneurial activity. Against this, Crouch depicts the institutional entrepreneur, 'looking for chances to change and innovate' (p. 37), and 'casting around for elements of institutions that they could recombine in unusual ways at opportune moments in order to produce change'.

The waste and redundancy left by past institutional changes provide the potential raw material of future transformations. Under conditions of uncertainty and exogenous shock, this can also serve to increase the resilience of socio-economic systems, by providing a rich and diverse range of institutional materials from which responses to those shocks may be built. Also of potential interest are the institutions and modes of governance that are being used by neighbours – and which might be borrowed and adapted (pp. 91–3).[5]

Nevertheless, the entrepreneurial activity that Crouch celebrates can also be deployed to reinforce existing inequalities and stasis. Lieberson (1987) argues that whatever processes of inequality operate, and whatever countervailing policies are introduced, purposeful actors will probe for alternative macro-dynamics that can defend their positions. One of his main illustrations is drawn from the area of social mobility. He takes racial inequalities in the US, in schooling and in occupational destinations. Any success in reducing those educational inequalities is unlikely to reduce corresponding inequalities in occupational outcomes, because more advantaged groups are likely to switch to other institutional means to sustain their position. This is a positional struggle, in which 'whites will give blacks as little as they can', consistent with the need 'to maintain the system and avoid having it overturned'. The means used to pursue this goal 'may however be highly variable and . . . modified by the idiosyncratic history of that setting'. They are also fraught with uncertainty (pp. 189–91).

In significant respects Lieberson is a precursor of complexity analysis applied to the social sciences. Throughout his study, he is at pains to argue that it is rare for a single causal process to be in operation; 'no equilibrium is really possible between the different causal forces'; there is only a 'constant flux' (p. 190). Lieberson is alerting us to the contingent and labile nature of these causal connections and the cascades of larger reconfiguration to which they may be subject, as a result of policy interventions that may have a narrower and more specific focus.

Social actors draw purposefully from macro-level

How shall we think of the 'macro-level' – and its relationship to the micro-level? We recalled earlier that for much of sociology – what Dawe (1970) calls the 'sociology of order' – the macro-level is seen in terms of the constraints that it imposes on the micro-behaviour of individual actors. From the moment we are born, we are confronted by an array of institutions into which we are socialised. We have also, however, pointed to a range of sociologists and those influenced by the 'complexity' literature for whom the macro 'emerges' from the micro and is then purposefully and endlessly re-woven.

In this unfolding drama the macro-level has a three-fold significance. First, it is from this macro-level that new social actors emerge, with their own powers, connections, resources and forms of organisation, ready for the fray. Macro encompasses potential allies and support networks among whom they can find a place of shelter; and from amid whose interstices they can venture forth and discover new opportunities for enterprise. However, it also encompasses predators waiting to pounce.

Second, macro is a reservoir of resources that social actors can combine and deploy in new ways. It makes available tools, skills and capacities that they can draw down and mobilise. It provides anchorage points for leverage, by which they can seek to change the world in which they live. It is the scrapyard of *bricolage* which they can plunder; and to which they can relegate the casualties and dross of previous rounds of positional struggle. Macro provides conventions and routines and a store of settled knowledge. It offers alternative institutional venues within which social actors can interact and a library of possible rules and precedents which they can invoke. It makes available cultural myths, legitimating narratives, social identities, group affiliations and organisational paradigms. These enable social actors to cooperate, to secure compliance, to allocate obligations and entitlements and to justify or contest modes of domination. It serves as a 'distributed system' of information and expertise which social actors can tap. This includes 'mental models' of the alternative futures that may unfold under conditions of uncertainty (Simon, 1969; North, 1990; Holland, 1995).

Third, macro is an environment which selects – in an evolutionary sense – from among the myriad pressures for change that bubble up from below, as micro-actors probe for the transformative dynamics from which they can benefit. Here macro is better viewed as a dynamic ecosystem, rather than as a market equilibrium or a fixed structure of hierarchical differentiation. This is, for example, evident in the work of Allen (1997) on the dynamic evolution of cities; in Room's account of the knowledge economy (Room, 2011a: ch. 16); and in Abbott's work on the development of neighbourhoods and professions (Abbott, 1997, 2001).

Throughout this discussion, we have juxtaposed the micro and the macro. Nevertheless, as social actors probe the macro-dynamics of their society, it is important to recognise that they do so at all intervening scales, depending on the scope for action that is open to them: a few across the society as a whole, but most of them just in their local environment. Even those who act on a global stage will draw on resources from their immediate professional and personal networks, in their efforts to lever change. It is their skill in weaving together their strong and weak ties, their links to formal and informal organisations, their multiple affiliations and their network memberships, that will be crucial to these efforts (Granovetter, 1973; Perri 6, 1996), whether they are lone parents juggling the competing demands of family and work on a low income (Millar and Ridge, 2013), or the executives of global corporations (Kristensen and Zeitlin, 2005).

1.4 Self-organisation and the imposition of order

There is a substantial literature that vindicates a 'complexity' perspective on the 'emergence' of macro-regularities from micro-interactions. Nevertheless, individual actors also, to some degree, make and impose their own order. There is a dynamic and evolving 'dance', between the self-organisation that may 'emerge' at the macro-level and the efforts of particular strategic actors to impose organisation and direction of their own. Nor does this refer only to the most powerful social, political and economic actors. Albeit on very different scales, we all bring our purposive actions to bear on the self-organising patterns that arise from myriad interactions across our society.

The 'dance' between self-organisation and the efforts of particular strategic actors applies not least to the analysis and development of public policy. Here we take two illustrations.[6]

Economic development

For some writers on complexity, including those influenced by Hayek, modern societies are over-regulated by the State and must be 'liberated' so that they can self-organise (Parker and Stacey, 1994). For Hayek himself, capitalism is a self-organising system and, as Desai and Ormerod (1998: 1431) summarise, 'the complex interaction of individual agents implies, for example, that government intervention is not needed to revive the economy in a depression. The natural rhythms of the system itself ensure that a recovery takes place'.

It can, however, be argued that leaving markets to self-organise may produce social consequences – in terms of social inequality and polarisation, for example – that undermine social consent and threaten a backlash against the very market institutions on which prosperity is said to depend (Polanyi, 1944). Keynes in particular doubted whether – to use the language of complex systems – a modern economy could self-organise at full employment of national resources and economic capacity, without the active intervention of the State. Only government could provide a framework of stable expectations within which capitalist entrepreneurs and their 'animal spirits' would flourish. Keynes thus saw the State as involved in a continuous dance with the market economy, in part by tuning monetary and fiscal policy, but also by direct intervention in terms of public expenditure and investment (Wagener and Drukker, 1986: ch. 4).

Expectations and confidence are irrelevant to the analysis of complex systems in the physical or biological world. In human societies, however – especially modern industrial societies, whose levels of economic activity depend on levels of investment – they are crucial in determining whether entrepreneurs act, or whether they sit on their funds, 'hunker down' and wait for better times. Public policy is thus of central interest, because of the role that it plays in the steering and management of society and economy, as a dynamic and open complex system.

Hirschman (1958) offers a not dissimilar perspective. He asks about the preconditions for economic development. The mainstream literature answers in terms of particular resources – natural resources, capital, entrepreneurs, etc. But, Hirschman points out, it proves difficult to agree empirically on which of these is key; and indeed, once development gets going, somehow they all fairly readily appear.

He, therefore, offers an alternative view. What seems to matter much more than any particular resource are the 'interlocking vicious circles' that hold development back; and, in contrast, the 'upward spirals' that can bring forth all the resources that are needed. The focus must, therefore, be not on the resources themselves but on the 'essential dynamic and strategic aspects of the development process' (Hirschman, 1958: 6). He adds that many of these resources may be latent rather than immediately available. They lie 'hidden, scattered or badly utilised' (p. 5): *bricolage* which can, however, with a little ingenuity, be adapted to new uses. Development depends on mobilising and combining these purposefully, but also in a spirit of experimentation: trying out different makeshift adaptations and finding which ones will work – and maybe even work well. It is this capacity to mobilise and combine, adapt and redeploy, that is the real determinant of development.

From this he infers that it is quite insufficient for governments to adopt a hands-off policy: backwardness and stagnation will be the inevitable result. But what is also inappropriate is to embrace a strategy of 'balanced growth', hoping to make simultaneous progress across all sectors to which the country in question aspires. Instead, Hirschman argues for development through a succession of 'imbalances', with each inducing a new phase of energetic investment. 'If the economy is to be kept moving ahead, the task of development policy is to maintain tensions, disproportions and disequilibria' (p. 66). This is a form of 'critical path analysis', which insists that the best path between two points is not necessarily a straight line. This, again, involves government in watching how the wider economy is blindly organising itself; taking specific measures to develop sectors which will generate the strategic 'upward spirals' which are needed; and nurturing those dynamic synergies as they unfold.

Social mobility

As we have seen, Lieberson examines patterns of social mobility in the US: in particular, racial inequalities in occupational achievement. He depicts a race between government, taking measures to promote equality, and white parents, seeking to defend their positions.

Goldthorpe offers a not dissimilar account of the stable pattern of class inequalities in social mobility to be found across western industrial societies over much of the last hundred years. He points to pressures from those who are more advantaged, seeking to promote the life chances of their own children (Erikson and Goldthorpe, 1993: 368–9, 393–7). If it had not been for the social and educational policies of the post-war period, these pressures would probably have exacerbated the inequalities in relative mobility chances: but with those policies, there has been stability of mobility inequalities (Goldthorpe, 1980: 275; Erikson and Goldthorpe, 1993: 368).

How are we to explain this contingent balance – bearing in mind Lieberson's counsel that 'no equilibrium is really possible between the different causal forces'?

Consider first the strategies of those in the more advantaged social classes. Faced with the widening intrusion of working-class families into traditionally middle-class institutions (selective schools, white collar and professional occupations), as egalitarian policies by the State take effect, we might posit a 'tolerance threshold' to such intrusion. Here more advantaged families bestir themselves in outflanking strategies, whose effect will be to block – or at least constrain – existing access routes, as used by working-class families, and to create new institutional by-passes that the more advantaged expect to reserve for themselves. There is plenty of empirical evidence of such efforts by more advantaged families (Lauder and Hughes, 1999: ch. 5; Ball, 2003: chs 4–6; Power et al., 2003: ch. 11; Swift, 2003; Smithers and Robinson, 2010).

Consider on the other hand the State, faced with the persisting efforts of the more advantaged to block or at least constrain working-class access routes. Here we might similarly posit a critical threshold in such blockages, at which the State bestirs itself, to limit the by-passes that the advantaged have developed for their offspring. Such strategies may be rather limited in their scope (scholarships for working-class children to go to private schools); or they may be more general and wide-ranging (common schools for all).

Here is a dynamic and evolving 'dance' between the State and social groups who dispose of different degrees of power and advantage. Here are two forms of agency, each aroused when a tolerance threshold is reached, and each producing a cascade of wider change. Pierson notes that it is close to such thresholds, when just a few valued positions are still vacant, that the competition among those poised to occupy them will increase in dramatic and non-linear fashion (Pierson, 2004: 83). Such effects encourage the use of a model of discontinuous change, with 'punctuated equilibria'.

As an example, Pierson points to models of avalanches in the physical sciences. One such model is Bak's 'self-organised criticality' (Bak, 1997). This he illustrates by means of an avalanche, not unlike the example we took from the hills of Svalbard. His model has also been applied to a wide range of physical, biological and social processes. Room (2011b) has shown how this model can capture the 'contingent' balance in social mobility in industrial societies. Again, however, this must be understood by reference to the political economy of the societies in question.[7]

1.5 Transformative realism

In this chapter, we assess the potential contribution of the literature on complex systems to some of the core questions and puzzles within social science. As well as the self-organisation that may 'emerge', individual actors, to some degree, make and impose their own order. This involves the negotiation of meanings and entitlements and obligations, and positional struggles within societies characterised by great inequalities of power and advantage. If social science is to take inspiration from the complexity literature, it must do so having full regard to the political economy of the social world.

This distinction between the natural and the social sciences must be held centre-stage. A complexity perspective applied to human societies must, to this extent, diverge from its origins in the natural and informational sciences if it is to illuminate the dynamics of those societies in their own specific terms. But rather than seeing this as an unwelcome complication, it should be seen as clarifying the way in which a complexity perspective can enrich social science.

In this section we consider some of the broad methodological implications of this position in terms of theory-building, modelling and empirical analysis.

Theory-building

If we are to explain natural or social phenomena, it is not enough to measure them, organise the resulting data into a statistical model and demonstrate that the coefficients of the model are robust and significant. One reason is that for non-linear systems, conventional statistical models have limited applicability (see also Chapter 3). In addition, however, there is a strong tradition within the philosophy of science which insists that explanation must include theory-building: that is, an account of the underlying processes which generate the phenomena in question, set within a more general conceptual scheme. This is the 'realist' tradition, which scholars such as Harré have championed during the last half-century, in relation to both natural and social science (Harré, 1972; Harré and Secord, 1972: ch. 4).

Harré places 'generative mechanisms' or processes at the centre of any scientific theory and explanation. The cause is not merely antecedent to the effect (as stressed by J. S. Mill): it generates it, whether by biochemical, physical, social or other processes. These 'causal powers' are, however, typically activated only in particular circumstances: it is the task of the scientist to lay bare these contingencies (Harré, 1972: 121). Explosives such as gunpowder and dynamite provide the example that Harré frequently cites. The chemical composition of the explosive provides the capacity or power to explode: but whether it does so or not depends on such factors as the absence of damp, the presence of oxygen, the ambient temperature, etc. Causal analysis of generative processes aims to reveal such contingencies.

Many social scientists have taken their lead from Harré. Thus, for example, Pawson (2006) offers a 'realist' critique of orthodox approaches to evidence-based policy-making, that rely on randomised control trials to produce generally applicable findings about the effectiveness of particular medical or social interventions. He points instead to the many contingencies which unlock, limit or modify the potential of such interventions and which shape their effects. The scientific task is to disentangle these contingencies and understand how the intervention works under various combinations of these circumstances.

This still leaves Pawson focusing primarily on the individual intervention – whether gunpowder or a new pharmaceutical product or a social policy programme – and unpicking the contingent factors that activate or inhibit its impact. Policy interventions are not isolated, however: they are launched into a crowded world. Nor are their forerunners merely the detritus of policy enthusiasms long forgotten; in many cases their champions are still at work, seeking to broaden their scope and to colonise the landscape onto which any new policy is launched. Nor is it just a matter of what combination of policies co-habit a given landscape. What can also matter is the order in which they are introduced. Sequence and timing are important: change them, and the ways in which they shape each other will also change (see also Chapter 7).

Policy interventions and their potentialities are not fixed, in the way that the chemical composition of gunpowder is fixed. On the contrary, the identity, the potentialities and the impact of any intervention are contingent on the various synergies that it develops – or fails to develop – with other interventions; and on the ways that those affected lever it to their own particular ends. We are, so to speak, interested not in gunpowder per se, but in the weapons technologies of which it is no more than a component, and whose potentialities, far from fixed, are the stuff of arms races. This is an *evolutionary* version of realism. The focus is still on generative processes, but these are now located not so much within individual interventions, but rather in the synergies that develop *among* these interventions and their stakeholders, as they co-evolve.

To use the term 'evolutionary' perhaps holds risks of misunderstanding. Evolution by natural selection is a blind process. In human societies in contrast, people probe, experiment and learn. They hope to discover dynamic synergies among the technologies and institutions of their world, which they can purposefully re-weave and direct to their own advantage. They strive thereby to develop their understanding and their capacities; their control over their lives; their positional advantage and leverage. This brings interests and power and politics centre-stage. We will, therefore, refer to this perspective as *transformative realism*.

We referred earlier to the 'downward causation' that develops within Schelling's model, as racial segregation 'emerges'. Biological co-evolution involves similar 'downward causation', as the dynamic synergies it discovers come progressively to dominate the ecosystems in question, limiting the scope for other species to thrive or even rendering them extinct. In human societies, social actors search purposefully for dynamic synergies which can similarly allow them to dominate the struggle for positional advantage. This is a generative process located not at the level of the individual actor, but in the leverage which such actors are able to exert on those emergent macro-level dynamics. To analyse and understand this leverage is the central task of social science research.[8]

The focus, therefore, must be not on the individual social actor or policy intervention, but on the dynamic interactions that develop among them and the contingent blockages on the exercise of their powers. In human affairs those blockages are constructed institutionally and historically: any realist account of potentialities created, unlocked or closed down is an account of this contingent historical and political struggle.[9] It must also recognise that different institutional arrangements will mean different potentialities released, as different institutional rules are invoked (see, for example, Etzioni, 1961; Ostrom, 1990). This is why it is important to root the analysis of generative processes within an explicitly institutionalist framework. This is a central task of this book.[10]

Models and empirical data

Ontology must precede epistemology and theory must drive method, not vice versa. Lieberson (1987) is therefore critical of much quantitative sociological research, notwithstanding the sophisticated forms of correlation and regression analysis that it offers. He questions the readiness of researchers to take the regression coefficients that emerge from such analysis as 'speaking for themselves' – and enabling them to adjudicate, on the basis of the variance they explain, as to the importance of different explanatory variables (ch. 5). Against this, he argues that it is only by reference to a specific theoretical question that we can make sense of the variables involved and assess their joint influence on the 'dependent variable' in question. These theoretical questions, we have just argued, must in turn be addressed by reference to the generative processes of the phenomena in question.

The complexity literature offers a range of models of non-linear change that illuminate the generative processes in which transformative realism is interested. At the start of this chapter we took examples of open complex systems from both the physical and the biological world. The hills of Svalbard – with their avalanches and striations – can be modelled as a process of 'punctuated equilibrium': what Bak, in one of the classic texts of complexity writing, refers to as 'self-organised criticality' (Bak, 1997).

As a second example, we took the evolutionary and co-evolutionary dynamics of the biological world. Here is a rich modelling literature on which a complexity-informed social science can draw (Crutchfield and Schuster, 2003; Solé and Bascompte, 2006). Such models will be an important point of reference in Chapter 3 of this book. Closely related are models of networks and their evolution: and the weaving of new connections between the elements of a system and its wider environment, to produce a novel dynamic (Room, 2011a: ch. 11).

In subsequent discussion, we have used Schelling's model of residential segregation. This is a simple model, but one which illustrates well how 'micro' emerges from 'macro' in non-linear ways and with counter-intuitive results.

The complexity literature has a wide range of other non-linear models, upon which social science may also usefully draw (Ball, 2004; Room, 2011a). These provide dynamic ideal types of non-linear change that can be used to illuminate the empirical social world. They may not allow precise prediction of the sort to which linear regression models typically aspire. They do, however, reveal the 'tipping points' and 'bifurcations' that follow from different values of the 'control parameters' or 'replicator dynamics' which generate that macro-behaviour

(Room, 2011a: ch. 9; Colander and Kupers, 2014: ch. 4). True, each model has its limitations, but that is the case with any ideal type.

Such models of non-linear change have become much more available, with the arrival of computational simulation. In general, however, they suffer from two limitations (Boero and Squazzoni, 2005; Room, 2011a: ch. 13; Byrne and Callaghan, 2014: ch. 7). First, the models have much to say about the emergence of macro from micro, much less about the institutional and political settings within which this emergence develops and the relations of power and compliance that interactions involve. This is a precondition for understanding the political alternatives to the present order of things.

Second, those who have elaborated computational models often fail to ground them empirically. Now, however, the same computational capacity that allows such modelling may also offer scope for the analysis of real time 'big data'. This may in the coming years enable researchers to identify empirically the self-reinforcing processes of emergence that can develop in social contexts and the alternative trajectories that they take under different conditions (Mayer-Schonberger and Cukier, 2013).

Variables, actors and systems

Social science comes in many varieties. They differ not least in the place they give to variables, actors and systems – and the relationships among them. This will also be a concern of this book.

The chapter began with systems, both closed and open, and their interacting elements. It took inspiration from the literature on complex systems and their capacity to 'self-organise', and it asked how far these insights could be extended from the natural to the social sciences. It took note of the efforts by complex system scholars to develop models and explanations of the non-linear macro-dynamics of such systems: it argued, however, the need to take account also of purposive actors, imposing order of their own on the social arrangements with which they found themselves faced. This is a continuing theme of this book.

To repeat, we have stressed the role of purposive actors in shaping such system dynamics. Agency and self-organisation are locked in an endless dance. But how is such action to be conceptualised? And in what ways does this provide a distinctive vantage point for critically reviewing the broad range of accounts of social action that we find in the social science literature? In subsequent chapters we challenge in particular the rational action literature and economic behaviourism: and we argue instead for our notion of 'agile action'.

Complex systems exhibit non-linear dynamics: the form that these take typically depends on the control parameters or variables of the system. However, much of the social world can be quite well-described in linear terms and social science offers a powerful array of technically sophisticated methods for modelling linear systems, in terms of independent and dependent variables. Chapter 3 is concerned with the limits of such approaches and seeks to articulate a clear non-linear alternative: an alternative on which subsequent chapters can then draw.

Variables we can measure. Actors we can interrogate, as to the rationale they may be able to provide for their actions. Non-linear systems we can study for their macro-dynamics, their bifurcations and the macro-configurations they take. In general, as social scientists, we must find a place for all three in our work: just how we do this goes to the heart of whatever social science we embrace.

1.6 Conclusion

The order and regularities of social life may attest in part to the self-organisation of society as a complex system, but they attest no less to the exercise of power, and the success of some social actors in negotiating or imposing that order on others. This brings interests and power and politics centre-stage: complexity analysis must be combined with institutional analysis and political economy (Room, 2011a).

The transformative macro-dynamics of the social world mean that there are multiple possible futures. This evokes a struggle, as different actors seek to limit such futures to those which will give them security and positional advantage. The range of possible futures is, however, obscure. Their demystification is central to the task of sociology (Berger, 1974), but this is always partial and slanted.

This should inform the analysis and development of public policy. It is not enough to look to the economy's self-organising propensities. Civility does not 'self-organise', it must be politically constructed, and we cannot escape the social and political choices of our time.

Notes

1 There is a range of good texts for the general reader which can be consulted for elaboration of the exposition offered here (Waldrop, 1992; Buchanan, 2000; Johnson, 2001; Ball, 2004; Boulton et al., 2015). Applications to social science include Jervis (1997), Byrne and Callaghan (2014). An example of some of the 'softer' strands of complexity writing in cultural studies is Cilliers (1998).
2 It is then possible to consider how far these physical processes can be captured – and further illuminated – in terms of the laws of thermodynamics and the production of entropy. That, however, we leave to the physicists (Stewart, 2003).
3 Physicists and biologists debate how far these biological processes can be understood by reference to physical entropy (Martyushev and Seleznev, 2006). There is also a debate as to whether self-organisation in both the physical and the biological worlds can be understood in terms of 'information', considered as a more generic counterpart to entropy (Shannon and Weaver, 1949). This, however, we leave to the physicists, the biologists and the information scientists.
4 For an easy introduction to Schelling's model and its simulation, see https://ccl.northwestern.edu/netlogo/
5 A closely parallel account of entrepreneurial actors is offered by Potts (2000), albeit focused on technological rather than institutional innovation.
6 One of the mathematical physicists to whom we referred at the outset was Ian Stewart. One of his interests is in the design of control systems for complex systems in engineering and medicine. These involve precisely the dance that will be described here: between the self-organisation of a complex system and the intervention, more or less

frequent by a human agent, so as to tune and steer how that system develops (Stewart, 1997: ch. 15). Or as Scott (1998: 327) describes this interaction: 'Each prudent, small step, based on prior experience, yields new and not completely predictable effects that become the point of departure for the next step.'

7 More simply, the strategies of the more advantaged households might be modelled as in Schelling, with those households vacating educational and professional arenas where too many of their neighbours are working class; meanwhile the State periodically takes action aimed at restoring the random distribution of households to those arenas which are in danger of becoming no-go zones as far as the working-class is concerned. In order to explore such possibilities, again see https://ccl.northwestern.edu/netlogo/

8 We earlier recalled Durkheim's treatment of the 'macro-level', as constituted by a variety of social forces that govern the frequency or rates of particular micro-actions and give them their stability. This has led to Durkheim being accused of reifying those forces and adopting an ahistorical functionalism. It is, therefore, worth noticing that his approach is more nuanced: 'Whenever certain elements combine and thereby produce, by the fact of their combination, new phenomena, it is plain that these new phenomena reside not in the original elements but in the totality formed by their union' (Durkheim, 1938: xlvii). Elder-Vass (2010) takes a similar position, when investigating the causal powers of entities in the physical, biological and social worlds. His interest is, like ours, in those generative mechanisms which operate only when the different elements of a system come together – and which are therefore to be seen as powers of that whole.

9 Marris (1996: ch. 7) offers a similar account of 'power as the mastery of contingencies rather than the accumulation of assets'.

10 We have presented our notion of 'transformative realism' in relationship to Harré, one of the founders of the 'realist' tradition in the philosophy of science. We have also referred to Pawson, a prominent contemporary practitioner, and to Elder-Vass. We do not attempt a more thorough and systematic commentary on other recent proponents of realism and 'critical realism' such as Bhaskar and Archer.

References

Abbott, A. (1997), 'Of Time and Space: The Contemporary Relevance of the Chicago School', *Social Forces*, 75(4): 1149–82

Abbott, A. (2001), *Time Matters: On Theory and Method,* Chicago: University of Chicago Press

Allen, P. (1997), *Cities and Regions as Self-Organizing Systems: Models of Complexity,* Amsterdam: Gordon and Breach Science Publishers

Bak, P. (1997), *How Nature Works: The Science of Self-Organized Criticality,* Oxford: Oxford University Press

Ball, P. (2004), *Critical Mass: How One Thing Leads to Another,* London: Heinemann

Ball, S.J. (2003), *Class Strategies and the Education Market: The Middle Class and Social Advantage,* London: RoutledgeFalmer

Berger, P.L. (1974), *Pyramids of Sacrifice: Political Ethics and Social Change,* Harmondsworth: Penguin

Boero, R. and F. Squazzoni (2005), 'Does Empirical Embeddedness Matter? Methodological Issues on Agent-Based Models for Analytical Social Science', *Journal of Artificial Societies and Social Simulation,* 8(4). <http://jasss.soc.surrey.ac.uk/8/4/6.html>

Boulton, J.G., P.M. Allen, and C. Bowman (2015), *Embracing Complexity: Strategic Perspectives for an Age of Turbulence,* Oxford: Oxford University Press

Bronowski, J. (1981), *The Ascent of Man,* London: Futura

Buchanan, M. (2000), *Ubiquity,* London: Wiedenfeld and Nicholson

Byrne, D. and G. Callaghan (2014), *Complexity Theory and the Social Sciences,* Abingdon: Routledge
Campbell, D.T. (1974), 'Downward Causation in Hierarchically Organised Biological Systems', in F.J. Ayala and T. Dobzhansky (eds), *Studies in the Philosophy of Biology: Reduction and Related Problems,* London: Macmillan: 179–86
Cilliers, P. (1998), *Complexity and Postmodernism,* London: Routledge
Colander, D. and R. Kupers (2014), *Complexity and the Art of Public Policy,* Princeton, NJ: Princeton University Press
Coleman, J. (1990), *Foundations of Social Theory,* Cambridge, MA: Harvard University Press
Crouch, C. (2005), *Capitalist Diversity and Change: Recombinant Governance and Institutional Entrepreneurs,* Oxford: Oxford University Press
Crutchfield, J.P. and P. Schuster, (eds) (2003), *Evolutionary Dynamics,* Oxford: Oxford University Press
Dawe, A. (1970), 'The Two Sociologies', *British Journal of Sociology,* 21(2): 207–18
Desai, M. and P. Ormerod (1998), 'Richard Goodwin: A Short Appreciation', *The Economic Journal,* 108: 1431–35
Dopfer, K. and J. Potts (2008), *The General Theory of Economic Evolution,* London: Routledge
Durkheim, E. (1897/1952), *Suicide,* London: Routledge and Kegan Paul
Durkheim, E. (1938), *The Rules of Sociological Method,* New York: Free Press
Elder-Vass, D. (2010), *The Causal Power of Social Structures: Emergence, Structure and Agency,* Cambridge: Cambridge University Press
Erikson, R. and J.H. Goldthorpe (1993), *The Constant Flux: A Study of Class Mobility in Industrial Societies,* Oxford: Clarendon
Etzioni, A. (1961), *Complex Organisations,* New York: Free Press
Flannery, T. (1994), *The Future Eaters,* New York: Grove Press
Goldthorpe, J.H. (1980), *Social Mobility and Class Structure in Modern Britain,* Oxford: Clarendon Press
Goldthorpe, J.H. (2007a), *On Sociology (2nd edition): Volume One: Critique and Program,* Stanford, CA: Stanford University Press
Goldthorpe, J.H. (2007b), *On Sociology (2nd edition): Volume Two: Illustrations and Retrospect,* Stanford, CA: Stanford University Press
Goldthorpe, J.H. and P. Bevan (1977), 'The Study of Social Stratification in Great Britain 1945–75', *Social Science Information,* 16(3–4): 279–334
Granovetter, M. (1973), 'The Strength of Weak Ties', *American Journal of Sociology,* 78: 1360–80
Harré, R. (1972), *The Philosophies of Science,* Oxford: Oxford University Press
Harré, R. and P.F. Secord (1972), *The Explanation of Social Behaviour,* Oxford: Blackwell
Hedström, P. (2005), *Dissecting the Social: On the Principles of Analytical Sociology,* Cambridge: Cambridge University Press
Hirschman, A.O. (1958), *The Strategy of Economic Development,* New Haven, CT: Yale University Press
Holland, J. (1995), *Hidden Order: How Adaptation Builds Complexity,* New York: Basic Books
Jervis, R. (1997), *System Effects: Complexity in Political and Social Life,* Princeton, NJ: Princeton University Press
Johnson, S. (2001), *Emergence: The Connected Lives of Ants, Brains, Cities and Software,* Harmondsworth: Penguin

Kaldor, N. (1985), *Economics without Equilibrium*, Cardiff: University College Cardiff Press

Kauffman, S.A. (1993), *The Origins of Order: Self-Organisation and Selection in Evolution*, Oxford: Oxford University Press

Kauffman, S.A. (1995), *At Home in the Universe: The Search for Laws of Self-Organisation and Complexity*, Harmondsworth: Penguin

Kristensen, P.H. and J. Zeitlin (2005), *Local Players in Global Games: The Strategic Constitution of a Multinational Corporation*, Oxford: Oxford University Press

Kuhn, T.S. (1970), *The Structure of Scientific Revolutions*, Chicago, IL: University of Chicago Press

Lauder, H. and D. Hughes (1999), *Trading in Futures: Why Markets in Education Don't Work*, Buckingham: Open University Press

Lieberson, S. (1987), *Making it Count: The Improvement of Social Research and Theory*, Berkeley: University of California Press

Marris, P. (1996), *The Politics of Uncertainty*, London: Routledge

Martyushev, L.M. and V.D. Seleznev (2006) 'Maximum Entropy Production Principle in Physics, Chemistry and Biology', *Physics Reports* 426, 1–45 doi:10.1016/j.physrep.2005.12.001:

Mayer-Schonberger, V. and K. Cukier (2013), *Big Data*, London: John Murray

Millar, J. and T. Ridge (2013), 'Lone Mothers and Paid Work: The "Family-work Project"', *International Review of Sociology*, 23(3): 564–77

Noble, D. (2006), *The Music of Life: Biology beyond Genes*, Oxford: Oxford University Press

North, D.C. (1990), *Institutions, Institutional Change and Economic Performance*, Cambridge: Cambridge University Press

Ostrom, E. (1990), *Governing the Commons: The Evolution of Institutions for Collective Action*, Cambridge: Cambridge University Press

Parker, D. and R. Stacey (1994), *Chaos, Management and Economics: The Implications of Non-Linear Thinking*, London: Institute of Economic Affairs

Pawson, R. (2006), *Evidence-Based Policy: A Realist Perspective*, London: Sage

Perri 6 (1996), *Escaping Poverty*, London: Demos

Pierson, P. (2004), *Politics in Time*, Princeton, NJ: Princeton University Press

Polanyi, K. (1944), *The Great Transformation*, New York: Rinehart

Popper, K.R. (1994), 'Models, Instruments and Truth: The Status of the Rationality Principle in the Social Sciences', in K.R. Popper (ed.), *The Myth of the Framework: In Defence of Science and Rationality*, London: Routledge: 154–84

Potts, J. (2000), *The New Evolutionary Microeconomics: Complexity, Competence and Adaptive Behaviour*, Cheltenham: Edward Elgar

Power, S., T. Edwards, G. Whitty, and V. Wigfall (2003), *Education and the Middle Class*, Buckingham: Open University Press

Room, G. (2011a), *Complexity, Institutions and Public Policy: Agile Decision-Making in a Turbulent World*, Cheltenham: Edward Elgar

Room, G. (2011b), 'Social Mobility and Complexity Theory: Towards a Critique of the Sociological Mainstream', *Policy Studies*, 32(2): 109–26

Schelling, T.C. (1978), *Micromotives and Macrobehaviour*, London: W.W. Norton

Scott, J.C. (1998), *Seeing like a State*, Newhaven, CT: Yale University Press

Shannon, C.E. and W. Weaver (1949), *The Mathematical Theory of Communication*, Urbana: University of Illinois Press

Simon, H.A. (1969), *The Sciences of the Artificial*, Cambridge, MA: MIT Press

Smithers, A. and P. Robinson (2010), *Worlds Apart: Social Variation Among Schools*, London: The Sutton Trust

Solé, R. and J. Bascompte (2006), *Self-Organization in Complex Ecosystems,* Princeton, NJ: Princeton University Press

Stewart, I. (1997), *Does God Play Dice? (2nd Edition),* Harmondsworth: Penguin

Stewart, I. (2003), 'The Second Law of Gravitics and the Fourth Law of Thermodynamics', in N.H. Gregersen (ed.), *From Complexity to Life: On the Emergence of Life and Meaning,* New York: Oxford University Press

Swift, A. (2003), *How Not to Be a Hypocrite: School Choice for the Morally Perplexed Parent,* London: Routledge

Wagener, H.-J. and J.W. Drukker, (ed.) (1986), *The Economic Law of Motion of Modern Society: A Marx-Keynes-Schumpeter Centennial,* Cambridge: Cambridge University Press

Waldrop, M.M. (1992), *Complexity: The Emerging Science at the Edge of Order and Chaos,* London: Viking

Weber, M. (1949), *The Methodology of the Social Sciences,* New York: Free Press

2 Evolution and the arts of civilisation[1]

2.1 Introduction

Evolutionary dynamics will be a significant point of reference for this book. This chapter, therefore, takes these as its focus, as the basis for much of the argument in subsequent chapters. However, it also recognises what in Chapter 1 we described as the ongoing 'dance', between evolution and the purposive interventions that social actors undertake, in order to impose organisation and direction of their own.

In 1898, Thorstein Veblen published his essay, 'Why is economics not an evolutionary science?' (Veblen, 1898: ch. 16). His argument was that economics *should* be an evolutionary science; but that it had not developed as such and was therefore inadequate to the tasks that it set itself (Hodgson, 1998).

Veblen's target was neoclassical economics. Walras, for example, had sought to model economics on the physics of his day and thus to make it a 'real science' (Beinhocker, 2007). For Walras, this meant taking market equilibrium as its analytical centrepiece. Veblen, however, argued that this left no place for learning and the growth of knowledge. He wanted economics instead to imitate evolutionary biology, incorporating endogenous processes of innovation and transformation.

Since Veblen wrote, his plea has not gone unanswered. Even if Walrasian economics retains its grip on the neoclassical mainstream, evolutionary economics has become a significant, if ill-defined, heterodoxy: including in recent times Hodgson, Loasby, Metcalfe, Potts and Beinhocker. Meanwhile other strands of heterodoxy – most obviously the Keynesian tradition – have reinforced Veblen's critique of 'equilibrium' thinking (Kaldor, 1985).

This chapter shares Veblen's doubts about the value of 'equilibrium', as the taken-for-granted analytical heart of economics, or indeed any social science. Like Veblen, it finds in evolutionary science a more appropriate analytical inspiration, with learning and the growth of knowledge centre-stage. Nevertheless, just how evolutionary ideas should be applied to the social world is by no means obvious; nor is the relationship between evolution and politics and public policy. It is with these questions that this chapter is concerned.

2.2 Darwin's journey reversed

Darwin (1859) offered an account of evolution through natural selection. The scarcity of food relative to the available population provokes an unending Malthusian competition for life, a 'struggle for existence'. However, in each generation some offspring embody new 'variations' which enable them to thrive and reproduce with greater success within their particular environment. (In modern Darwinism, we understand these variations in terms of genetic recombinations and mutations.) These superior varieties then become progressively better-represented in successive generations. It is from these blind population dynamics – 'blind' in that there is no overall intent or purpose – that the differentiation and adaptation of species arise.

Those who champion evolutionary ideas are by no means agreed on just *how* they should be applied to the social world. For Dawkins, it is a matter of understanding social dynamics by reference to the demands of biological evolution. Thus, for example, it is by reference to the 'selfish gene' that we may understand the evolution of cooperation and altruism in societies (Dawkins, 1976). His account of the evolution of cultural 'memes', on the analogy of the evolution of genes, likewise makes social evolution subservient to the biological template. In contrast, Odling-Smee (Odling-Smee *et al.*, 2003) is a biologist who recognises the distinctive role played in human societies by cultural transmission, whose effects can, indeed, quite overwhelm those of biological selection.

Evolutionary economists such as those mentioned earlier go further, leaving no place at all in their analysis for biological selection.[2] New 'variations' emerge from the 'animal spirits' and inventiveness of entrepreneurs, in what Schumpeter (1934) described as 'swarms of innovation'. In Darwinism, it is the genetic legacy of a species that is reworked; in evolutionary economics, it is the technological and institutional legacy of the society. Political scientists such as Streek and Thelen (2005), in their account of institutional evolution, similarly treat the creativity of institutional entrepreneurs as the source of new variations.

Amid this variety, the present chapter insists on a quite specific point of departure: *we must start by reversing Darwin's journey*. Darwin's account began with his observation of husbandry and artificial selection, as practised by the pigeon breeders and horticulturalists he knew, and indeed by Darwin himself on his estate (Darwin, 1859: ch. 1). The breeder or horticulturalist looked out for novel characteristics in the offspring of each new generation that would better meet his or her requirements. These superior varieties were then selected for breeding, so as to combine and progressively accentuate these advantages. From here Darwin made the mental leap to posit 'natural selection', with the harsh struggle for scarce sustenance culling the less fit as rigorously – albeit over a much longer time period – as the breeder or horticulturalist. In adapting his model of evolution and natural selection to human societies, we move back into the practices of active husbandry from which Darwin began.

These are the arts of civilisation. Instead of blind adaptation of a population to different environments, they involve reflection, learning, experimentation, collaboration and the growth of knowledge. This is true of the husbandry of pigeons and livestock and plants: it is also true of the 'cultivation' by entrepreneurs of new technologies and institutions. Husbandry here reworks the technological and institutional legacy – as distinct from the genetic legacy – in hope of producing variants more suited to human purposes.

This chapter is therefore concerned less with natural selection and evolution, more with the breeder and artificial selection. Nevertheless, reversing Darwin's journey involves more than simply shifting from blind and impersonal selection in the wild to the considered and intentional selection practised by the horticulturalist or the entrepreneur. Artificial and natural selection have a more complex interrelationship.

- The horticulturalist or pigeon breeder is never entirely separate from the wild, the arena of natural selection. On the one hand, it was from the wild that varieties that appeared of interest for human purposes were originally drawn; the wild continues as a source of further novelties, which the breeder can hardly afford to ignore. (Think, for example, of the efforts by corporations to identify – and even to patent – genetic novelties in remote corners of the earth that may prove commercially exploitable.) On the other hand, many of the species that human activity has selected and cultivated can survive and thrive only insofar as they are protected from the wild and its processes of natural selection (Pollan, 2003, 2006: ch. 2). In short, *artificial and natural selection are forever competing for turf.*
- The artificial selection of pigeons and plants involves more than the breeder's attentive observation of unusual characteristics in each new generation, and the selection of some for further breeding. Beyond the breeder, what is also involved is selection by the market – by the purchasers of these novel breeds. It is ultimately the preferences of consumers – not of the breeder – that dictate which novelties survive and thrive.

  This is true not only of plant and stock breeders, reworking the genetic legacy; it applies to entrepreneurs more generally, reworking the technological legacy of their society to produce novelties that may better serve human purposes (Potts, 2000; Beinhocker, 2007). These entrepreneurs may, of course, seek through advertising and branding to shape consumer preferences. They can draw on their experience and their 'mental models' of the future in trying to anticipate market trends. Nevertheless, how a given technological innovation will fare – and how it may interact or be combined with other technologies and institutions – can never be entirely foreseen.

  In short, therefore, artificial selection *proposes* new variants: but it is processes of differential selection through the market that *dispose*; and these may be just as collectively 'blind' and devoid of overall intent as the processes of natural selection that drive speciation in the wild.
- Just as entrepreneurs bring forward technological novelties, institutional innovators bring forward new institutional forms (Pierson, 2004; Crouch, 2005; Streek and Thelen, 2005). These may involve new combinations of the institutional past, as well as institutional forms borrowed from elsewhere. Many may be ignored, but some will be adopted and adapted by social actors across the society. This again is selection by population dynamics.

  Some new institutional forms may be introduced because they enable particular new technologies to thrive (North, 1990). Think, for example, of e-commerce as a new institutional form, enabling the new information and communication technologies to flourish. However, another common aim of institutional entrepreneurs is to construct new lines of institutional differentiation in the population, so as to consolidate their positions of advantage. Think, for example, of patenting and copyright. Think also of the efforts of middle-class parents to capture the best schools and limit working-class access. Here institutional differentiation is not so much an impersonal and blind process of market dynamics, but in part at least *a struggle for positional advantage* within the population.

This then suggests a re-examination of the market itself, as a selection arena. Rather than blind population dynamics, selecting by reference to fitness for human purposes, the market must also, in part at least, be reconceptualised in terms of more powerful actors shaping technological and institutional change, so as to secure their positional advantage within that population.[3]

- Technological and institutional innovators practise what we earlier termed the 'arts of civilisation'. However, this is also a struggle for positional advantage, whose outcome may be anything but civil.

Darwin observes that 'we behold the face of nature bright with gladness' and its 'superabundance of food'; but we too easily overlook the concomitant destruction of life entailed by the incessant 'struggle for existence' (Darwin, 1859: 50). The same goes for human affairs and the struggle for positional advantage. If below the surface of nature's superabundance it is necessary to discern the struggle and destruction this entails, it is also necessary, below the order and regularities of social life, to discern *the exercise of power* by which these regularities are reproduced. If this is order, it is such only because some social actors have succeeded in negotiating or imposing that order on others.

Attempts to apply evolutionary models to the social world have in general neglected the exercise of power. By reversing Darwin's journey, taking account of artificial as well as natural selection, we bring power centre-stage.

- Darwin's gardener or pigeon breeder brought human purpose to the 'struggle for existence': influencing the variations that appear, selecting among them, protecting them, shaping the ensemble of flora and fauna which would make up the garden as a whole. In human affairs no less, fundamental choices of public policy and purpose are posed, as to the directions of change that citizens and policy-makers wish to cultivate, modifying the interests and power that drive the positional struggle. *This is husbandry of the social fabric, applying the arts of civilisation to society as a whole.* It is in these terms that the final section of this chapter will examine public policy.
- The arts of civilisation involve reflection, experimentation and the growth of knowledge. Human beings thereby produce or create themselves as a species (Bronowski, 1981).[4] *In producing themselves, however, human beings also produce the conditions of life for their fellow species.* Anthropogenic change is now a major feature of the selective environment to which other species must adapt, in their own struggle for existence (Le Page, 2011).[5]

Evolution and the arts of civilisation 35

We now examine in more detail what it means to 'reverse Darwin's journey', making artificial selection the vantage point from which we apply evolutionary models to technological and institutional change, but doing so with due regard for the complex interrelationship between artificial and natural selection – the 'dance' in which they are locked – that has just been outlined.[6] We pose three questions in turn:

1 How shall we conceive of human agents and their efforts to select from their institutional and technological legacy? How do they practise the discrimination that artificial selection involves?
2 How do human agents, by re-weaving their technological and institutional legacy, probe and unlock the potentialities of their world?
3 How shall we conceive of the 'struggle for existence' in which human actors are involved? How far does this involve a definition of fitness that still allows us to apply the insights of the evolutionary analogy?

In each case we then, like Veblen, consider what distinctive and critical vantage point this provides in relation to mainstream social science. By moving from artificial to natural selection, Darwin powerfully contested contemporary accounts of the natural order; we move from natural to artificial selection and critically contest prevailing accounts of the social order.

The chapter turns finally to the arts of civilisation as expressed in public policies.

2.3 Agile action: seeing what is new

Natural selection involves the transmission of genetic information between generations: information as to how organisms can successfully operate within different selective environments (Maynard Smith and Szathmary, 2000; Odling-Smee *et al.*, 2003). There is therefore no need for each generation to discover this for itself. This information is tested and revised in each generation. It is populations that thus evolve: individual organisms do not.

In some species organisms are also able to obtain information from other individuals during their lifetimes. This is the case with humans in particular, where cultural products and processes allow shared learning and the 're-blending' of that cultural inheritance by the young (Odling-Smee *et al.*, 2003: 258–9). Again, however, it is by taking as their starting point the wisdom of the ancients – as embodied in the tools, habits and conventions that they have left – that the young are best placed to experiment and advance the knowledge base.

It is by reference to this starting point that humans practise the discrimination that is involved in artificial selection: the first of the questions posed at the end of the previous section. They assess situations using standard templates, by reference to which they can make routine responses. These are search strategies using 'if-then' algorithms as a cognitive shortcut. Loasby (1999: chs 3, 8) locates this within the exigencies of human evolution. Survival required that the brain should be able quickly to recognise predators and prey, not that it should make careful comparisons of the costs and benefits of different strategies.

It is institutions and culture that carry these templates for survival (Douglas, 1986; Bowker and Star, 2002). There is, therefore, no need for each human to assess each situation by reference to the full range of possible behaviours (an immensely costly activity in terms of the energy and time involved). Instead, they can draw selectively from a shared inventory of templates and apply them to specific local situations. In general, the wisdom of the ancients is sufficient: in relation to the technologies and institutions that people employ (Bronowski, 1981: ch. 2), the foods that they eat (Pollan, 2006: ch. 16), the ways that they die (Kellehear, 2007). This is a second cognitive shortcut.

In times of change, these cultural templates may not suffice. However, humans not only learn from the past, they can also imagine a range of possible futures. They bring with them more or less well-articulated mental models of how their world will unfold under conditions of uncertainty. This is a third cognitive shortcut. It allows humans to innovate and to imagine the larger consequences that their innovations may set in motion: and thus not only to survive, but also to seize and wager on opportunities for future advantage.

Therefore, as well as applying the wisdom and habits of the ancients, the arts of civilisation involve identifying emerging situations of threat and opportunity, where this wisdom must be reworked for new circumstances. Indeed, it is precisely by applying the wisdom of the past that attention can be most effectively focused on the challenge of whatever is new. Even if we blaze new pathways, we keep one foot on the safe ground we know, while with the other we test and try out the new possibilities. In doing so, we contribute to the growth of knowledge and of our own skills and capacities (Bronowski, 1981: ch. 3).

In his critique of Walrasian economics, Veblen challenged its focus on rational economic man, with roots in hedonistic psychology. This went hand in hand with market equilibrium, as its analytical centrepiece, with neither leaving any place for learning and the growth of knowledge, nor indeed for processes of endogenous historical development. Against this, Veblen offered a view of human activity that gave pride of place to habits and conventions: seen not as the refuge of the irrational and thoughtless, but rather as the embodiment of the wisdom of the past, by reference to which novelties and inventions could most efficiently be crafted, and duly selected in terms of their fitness or relevance to human purposes. It is this view of habits and conventions that Veblen rightly sees as central to a Darwinian evolutionary perspective on technological and institutional change.

To some degree echoing Veblen, we pause to consider how the notion of human action elaborated here relates to more general debates about social action. Much has been written in recent years about the merits of rational choice and rational action theory in sociology, political science and economics (Coleman, 1990; Goldthorpe, 2000: ch. 3; Hedström, 2005). Our own approach is more nuanced. Following what has been said above, we may see much social action as involving pattern recognition and responses that Weber (1949) would have described not so much as rational but as 'habitual', made by reference to an inventory of templates and 'rules of thumb', encoded within social institutions.

It does not follow that all action and interaction is habitual. Faced with novel situations, uncertainty and turbulence, human actors deploy mental models as to how the world will unfold. This we may describe as 'agile' action (see also Chapter 4). Habitual action involves recognising a pattern and making a standard response. Agile action means reworking that pattern, having regard to conjectures as to how the world is likely to unfold. Between these two ideal types of action there is a dual connection. First, as we have seen, the cognitive economy in the former leaves maximum energy for the latter. Second, however, we must recognise that empirically, which matters are handled in which way is itself fluid. It is when actors detect anomalous patterns, including for example those that fall outside certain critical thresholds, that this alerts them to the need to make an agile response. These are typically situations that present opportunities or threats of major strategic significance. In short, what the if-then rules in this case prescribe is that the matter be removed from the if-then realm of the habitual. This is, therefore, an agenda forever in flux, and one that will vary greatly between actors, depending on their interests and the agility, resources and positional leverage of which they dispose. (For a somewhat parallel discussion, see Nelson and Winter (1982: ch. 5).)

This diverges from rational action theory, as normally articulated, in three respects. Rational action theory does not recognise the cognitive economies we have attributed to habitual action and the cultural wisdom those habits embody, freeing the energy and attention that can then be focused on the challenge of the new. Nor, therefore, does it recognise the connections we have just indicated between habitual and agile action. Second, it typically views the social actor as confronted with a given menu of options, carrying particular costs, benefits and consequences. Here, in contrast, we highlight the agile actor who, rather than taking that menu as given, actively seeks to reshape the rules of the institutional – and indeed the technological – landscape on which social interactions play out, precisely so as to change the options it offers (Dopfer and Potts, 2008: para. 3.2.1). Third, rational action theory treats the social actor as existing in an essentially timeless environment. Here, in contrast, we highlight the wisdom of the ancients and the path dependency of the habits and conventions with which we are endowed; and the uncertainty of the future, in face of which we can at best apply our mental models of how the world will develop, but always and irreducibly only as conjectures.[7]

Of course, we might decide to redefine rational action, so as to encompass this wider range of subjectively meaningful actions (Hedström, 2005: 62). It is after all 'rational' to be agile and to reshape the menu whenever possible, so as to make it more attractive (and irrational to ignore such possibilities, merely adjusting to whatever menu results from the contests of others). It is also 'rational' to adopt wherever possible simple if-then rules of habit, so as to reduce the energy required by careful calculation. Goldthorpe, for example, offers a discussion of the evolution of human cognitive architecture similar to that which we have discussed in relation to Loasby, with its 'simple, fast and frugal heuristics'; this however he continues to regard as being on a continuum with other forms of rationality (Goldthorpe, 2007: 180–1). Gilbert goes even further, seeing rational action as action according to any 'reasonable set of rules', as distinct from 'acting randomly or irrationally' (Gilbert, 2008: para. 1.3.5). Nevertheless, whatever terms are used, we must recognise this connected logic of habitual and agile action in an uncertain and shifting world, rather than just the rational assessment of benefits and costs in a static world.[8]

2.4 Combinatorial contingency: unlocking potential

We turn now to the second of the questions posed earlier in relation to 'reversing Darwin's journey'. How do human agents, by re-weaving their technological and institutional legacy, probe and unlock the potentialities of their society and their world? As in the previous section, we start with the Darwinian account of natural selection: from there we move back to the practices of active husbandry from which Darwin began.

Each generation of a population throws up new combinations of its genetic legacy. It is upon these variations that natural selection operates, allowing some to thrive more than others. Henceforth it is their genetic make-up that will be preponderant, within the species concerned. The direction of evolutionary development of a given species is however by no means random. The genetic legacy encodes past investments, which enable but also limit and channel subsequent development. History matters: evolution is path-dependent (Shubin, 2008).

Evolutionary journeys can be visualised as an adaptive walk across a fitness landscape (Kauffman, 1993). By combining elements of its genetic legacy in new ways, a species shifts its genotype (its position horizontally within Figure 2.1); it may thereby be able to increase its fitness, as measured by the height of the landscape. However, all species find themselves on landscapes that are more or less rugged, reflecting the afore-mentioned constraints and the path dependency of past development. There is, therefore, always the risk of getting caught on a low peak, unable to ascend further without costly descents into intervening valleys.

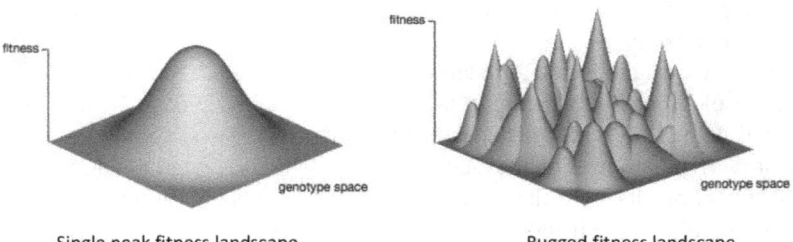

Single peak fitness landscape   Rugged fitness landscape

Figure 2.1 Fitness landscapes

No species makes its evolutionary journey in isolation. The fitness landscapes of different species are linked. They co-evolve. In some cases this is an antagonistic process, an 'arms race' between predator and prey species. In others it is a process of mutually beneficial adjustment, as for example between insects and flowering plants. The evolutionary journey of a given species, re-weaving its genetic legacy and unlocking its potentialities, is path-dependent therefore by reference not only to that legacy, but also to the ecosystems of which it has become part. It is on the contingent combination of this dual legacy that natural selection acts.[9]

Such journeys of evolutionary biology are slow, blind and without overall intent. The evolving genotype is passive. In contrast, the artificial selection practised by Darwin and his neighbours was active, rapid and intentional. The notion of an adaptive journey is here more than just metaphor, whether applied to pigeons or to technological and institutional innovations. It is in these terms that we now consider how human agents, by re-weaving their technological and institutional legacy, can probe and unlock the potentialities of their society and their world.

The journey starts with novelty or variation: new combinations of the technological and institutional legacy. Among evolutionary economists, Potts (2000) adopts just such a combinatorial ontology, applied to technologies for purposes of production. A similar ontology is evident in Crouch (2005), applied to institutions. Both writers highlight the role of entrepreneurs – whether in the realm of production or institutional governance – who rework these combinations and bring in new elements, so as better to achieve their purposes. Both of them also underline that in weaving these new combinations, entrepreneurs draw on the templates and practices of the past, but also deploy mental models of the uncertain future.[10]

Like the fitness landscapes of biological evolution and natural selection, technological and institutional innovation are strongly path-dependent. Past investments build capacity, interests and power in ways that will facilitate some future journeys, while blocking others. Here, however, in contrast to the evolutionary journeys of biology, human actors are forever on the lookout for opportunities deliberately to reshape those constraints and path dependencies.

Entrepreneurs experiment with combinations – we might say 'ecologies' – of technologies and institutions. They try to avoid the 'evolutionary catastrophes' of a 'low peak', an evolutionary *cul de sac*, or a fruitless arms race. Instead they hope to discover new co-evolutionary dynamics that will produce 'runaway' improvements from relatively modest investments. Such dynamics may entail co-evolution between different technologies; between new technologies and new markets; between new forms of industrial organisation and new systems of public regulation, etc. Thus do humans seek to reshape the contours of their fitness landscapes: exalting valleys, making the mountains low and the rough places plane. Whatever the mental models they deploy, however, both catastrophes and runaways may be difficult to spot until after the event.

To discover and nurture such dynamics is central to what we have called the arts of civilisation. It involves selective probing, trying out imaginative new combinations and discovering their potential, not randomly but by systematic testing and learning (Bronowski, 1981: chs 2–4). It involves decomposing the world into those parts that will for the moment be taken as given, as against those that will be reworked until their potential for runaway is exhausted. 'Exhaustion' here means not just that no further runaway is available; but also that the co-evolutionary dynamics that have produced these runaway improvements are routinised into standard operating procedures, habits and conventions. In other words, they are now part of the stock of traditional templates, well-honed tools and skills on which later-comers can draw.

This now provides a new vantage point – a new point of leverage – from which other components of the world can similarly be investigated. Nothing in our technological and institutional legacy is incontestable: nevertheless, the adaptive journey requires that we always keep one foot on solid and well-tried ground, even as the other tests out the new.[11] Again, however, the sequence of these steps – and of the arenas chosen for selective probing – is fateful for future directions of travel.

Darwin often repeats: '*Natura non facit saltum*' (nature makes no leaps). The adaptive walk of the evolutionary journey involves a succession of small-scale variations that slowly explore the contours of the fitness landscape, avoiding the risks involved in long-distance change. Nevertheless, as Darwin's successors have recognised, small steps can lead to discontinuous change, in the form of 'punctuated equilibria', with periods of stasis followed by larger-scale cascades of reconfiguration (Gould and Eldridge, 1977). In the social and economic world, the runaway changes to which we have referred can also have this character, with sudden cultural shifts and tipping points dramatically transforming the landscape. We may keep one foot on solid and well-tried ground, but in testing out the new, we may find that ground suddenly changing beneath our feet.

In the previous section, the arts of civilisation were discussed in terms of the relationship between habitual and agile action. Here we have discussed them in terms of the search for connections and co-evolutions that will yield runaway change. The art here consists in recognising these potential dynamics and making appropriate connections within a complex contingent structure. This perspective is what in Chapter 1 we referred to as 'transformative realism'.

If the arts of civilisation involve the exploration, development and testing of a complex contingent landscape, this takes us far from the notion of market equilibrium, the centrepiece of Walrasian economics and the target for Veblen's critique. As in the previous section, we finish by noticing some connections with more general debates in social science.

First, equilibrium analysis posits a system of variables and interrelationships, set in a larger context or environment, taken as 'given'. Negative feedback ensures stability when the system is disturbed. Competitive markets ensure the prevalence of such effects. Empirically, however, it is evident that positive feedback often predominates (Arthur *et al.*, 1997). Social and economic activities fatefully sculpt the surrounding context in ways that can be self-reinforcing. These are processes of 'cumulative causation' and they make for an 'economics without equilibrium'

(Kaldor, 1985; Toner, 1999). They arise not least because the social and economic actors in question actively seek them. This was of course central to the foregoing account of the quest for 'runaway' change.

Second, we follow Dawe (1970) in noticing two contrasting perspectives in social science. One highlights the 'problem of order' and sees individuals as simply adjusting to the changing social structures and circumstances in which they find themselves. This perspective resonates well with the equilibrium concerns of Walrasian economics. The other highlights the 'problem of control' and emancipation. It brings individual definitions of the situation centre-stage; as also therefore the contesting of such definitions, the strategies of action they inform and the social interactions – cooperative, competitive, conflictual – which ensue. Social systems here appear not as the locus of order but as the emergent outcome – to some extent unanticipated – of social interactions among myriad individuals. If this is order, it is so because some social actors have succeeded in negotiating or imposing that order on others, shaping the terms on which, for example, the economy 'self-organises' or different communities are empowered. This is, however, always provisional and contingent, in face of the ever-renewed struggle for control.

Finally, we have argued that what matters is the sequence in which combinations and connections are made and co-evolutions are set in motion – all serving to unlock potential or close it down, creating critical junctures, thresholds and tipping points. In like manner, Harré would have us think of causal processes as releasing or blocking potentialities (Harré, 1972: 121–2). Causal chains are also of political concern. They are constructed institutionally and historically. If they are complex and contingent, subject to cascades of reconfiguration, this is because they are forever being contested and reshaped, in the struggle for positional advantage. Harré's account of potentialities, critical thresholds and novel dynamics, can be read as much as an account of this historical and political struggle as a contribution to the philosophy of science.[12]

2.5 The positional struggle

We turn now to the third of the questions posed earlier in relation to 'reversing Darwin's journey'. How shall we conceive of the 'struggle for existence' in which human actors are involved? How far does this involve a definition of fitness that still allows us to apply the insights of the evolutionary analogy? We again start with the Darwinian account of natural selection, returning from there to the practices of active husbandry.

Natural selection is selection by population dynamics. It is those 'variations' that thrive and reproduce most vigorously that are progressively better-represented in successive generations. It is thus that they reveal – to us as intelligent observers – their superior 'fitness'. This is, of course, fitness in relation to the particular environment that the population in question occupies (both the physical environment and the encompassing ecosystem). Locally isolated populations in different environments will therefore select according to different criteria of fitness and they will progressively differentiate themselves into distinct subspecies (Darwin's finches in the Galapagos being the classic example).

Darwinian evolution is a blind process. Artificial selection, in contrast, is a deliberate human activity. Fitness is here something that human innovators attempt to judge *ex ante*, rather than just waiting for it to be revealed *ex post*.

What do we mean by 'fitness' in the context of artificial selection? In agriculture, we might refer to hardier strains of wheat, for example, that can thrive in colder climes or are more resistant to natural predators. As in the case of natural selection, it is if these strains survive and thrive with greater success that they demonstrate their superior fitness. Only the source of the variation differs. Rather different is the case of the pigeon bred for its speed of flight or elegance, or the apple for its taste: here it is the delight of the breeder or the customer that dictates which varieties of pigeons and apples will thrive. The customer is now the most important component of the selective environment.

Different again is the technological novelty that the entrepreneur brings to market. Here are no natural predators: the selection process is entirely within the market place of human consumers and their desires. Here, however, it is insufficient to assert that customer delight in different technological novelties – like customer delight in different apples – will dictate which varieties predominate. Technological novelties not only delight customers' hedonistic impulses, they also enable them to develop new systems of production and profit, to explore new runaways, to extend their power and their positional advantage.

As argued previously, this pursuit of positional advantage is even more evident when we turn from technologies to the evolution of institutions. New institutional forms bring new lines of differentiation in the population, consolidating the positions of some while excluding others, or else incorporating them – locking them in – on adverse terms. Instead therefore of blind population dynamics selecting by reference to the 'fitness' of different variations, powerful actors here actively shape technological and institutional change, as they struggle for positional advantage within that population.[13]

How then shall we think of 'positional advantage' within a population, driving artificial selection no less than the 'fitness' that drives natural selection (see also Chapter 5 below)?

Already in the previous section we saw that the entrepreneur is forever weaving new combinations of technologies and institutions, in hope of discovering co-evolutionary dynamics that will yield runaway improvements in position. This search – embodying as it does processes of reflection, learning and intentionality – is oriented to an uncertain future. It deploys mental models of how the changing world is liable to unfold. These models are, however, varied and provisional: different entrepreneurs are, therefore, likely to make different judgements of the future positional advantage that particular investments will bring.

Positional advantage can mean scope for profit-taking by bringing scarce and valued novelties to market. It can mean rent-taking by placing institutional restrictions on access to markets by competitors. It can involve 'first mover' privileges: the opportunity to have first shot at investigating and benefitting from new runaways (albeit this can be so risky that it is sometimes better to be a second mover). It can mean privileged access to processes of life chance distribution, by institutional arrangements that incorporate other population groups only on adverse terms. It can mean offloading the costs of uncertainty onto others. Above all, however, it means a protected and privileged vantage point within an uncertain future.

As in previous sections, our discussion of positional advantage and the arts of civilisation permits some comment on larger debates in social science, concerned with positional struggle. Hirsch (1977), for example, provides a simple but influential account of positional goods and the 'positional economy'. The distribution of its fruits – unlike those of the 'material economy' – is a zero-sum game. To some degree at least, educational credentials have this character. Hirsch sought clear principles – not just in theoretical terms but as a matter of practical politics – as to the distributional basis for such positional goods, so as to avoid a self-defeating competition (see also Chapter 5 below).

Other writers go beyond Hirsch, highlighting the ever-intensifying character of this positional struggle. First mover advantage allows actors to block developments they oppose; to build resilience; to maintain their own freedom of manoeuvre, keeping others guessing as to what they will do next; to offload uncertainty onto others and to destabilise them so that they cannot mount a challenge (Marris, 1996; Pierson, 2004). The struggle for positional leverage is, therefore, *a struggle to occupy the future*: to ensure that come what may, tomorrow is likely to turn out well for the protagonists in question, allowing them to weave their own futures, rather than being obliged to move to the rhythms of others (Abbott, 2001: 247). This is why, as Keynes for example observes, the accumulation of wealth is often not so much for eventual consumption, it is for some indefinitely distant date, to ensure a place in the sun, whatever the future disposition of the world (Tily, 2007: 142).

We return finally to Veblen. In the essay that provided our starting point, Veblen may not explicitly examine the pursuit of positional advantage, still less does he examine how this sits within an evolutionary perspective on economic development. Nevertheless, in other of his writings that theme moves centre-stage. In particular, Veblen provides a scathing account of the super-rich of his day, the 'leisure class' (Veblen, 1899). Their conspicuous consumption advertises their positional advantage, reinforces their social and economic distance from the larger society and provides ever-renewed symbols of the good life, to which that larger society is enjoined to aspire. This critique is echoed by James Galbraith (2009: chs 7, 9), the most prominent contemporary exponent of this robust tradition. He describes the modern-day counterpart to the leisure class as 'predatory': a new class of oligarchs devoted to rapacious looting (see also Akerlof and Romer, 1993).

When we described the positional struggle which artificial selection entails, we touched both on technological novelties, whetting the delights of customers but also enabling them to build new systems of production and profit, and on processes of institutional differentiation, by which the positional advantage of some is reinforced, while others are incorporated on adverse terms. It is in these terms that Galbraith depicts the current economic order and, more particularly, the financial crisis of recent years. On the one hand, new financial products and services were invented to cater for the different expectations, time horizons and risk stances of different market actors. Nevertheless, what is also well-documented is that some of these new instruments were designed to evade the regulators (notably their rules on the capital base that banks must maintain on their lending) and by their complexity to conceal the riskiness of the assets which they represent (notably in the case of sub-prime lending) (Soros, 2008: ch. 4; Brummer, 2009; Tett, 2009: ch. 2). At the same time the development of these instruments permitted predation on the major institutions of society – corporations, banks, housing finance, education and health, pensions – for purposes of private gain at public expense. The result has been adverse incorporation and looting of the most vulnerable.

2.6 Policy science and the evolutionary legacy

Veblen's essay of 1898 provided our point of departure. There Veblen argued that economics *should* be an evolutionary science; but that it had not developed as such, and was therefore not fit for purpose. We now pose a parallel question: 'What sort of policy science is implied by this evolutionary legacy?' The answer is two-fold.

First, we share Veblen's doubts about 'equilibrium' and 'rational action' as the taken-for-granted heart of economics, or indeed any social science. Instead, and again like Veblen, we find in evolutionary science a more appropriate analytical inspiration, which brings learning and the growth of knowledge centre-stage. We have however insisted that in applying evolutionary ideas to the social world, it is necessary to 'reverse Darwin's journey' and take artificial rather than natural selection as the analytical starting point.

Nevertheless, as we saw in section 2.2, the practice of artificial selection can hardly be entirely separate from the wild. A new variety of plant developed by the horticulturalist will succumb to the competitive pressures of natural selection, unless it is kept in a wholly artificial environment. The entrepreneur who develops new technologies or institutions is likewise at the mercy of blind population dynamics across the wider society, as different population groups adopt and adapt – or else ignore – the novelties he or she has brought forth, and connect – or fail to connect – them with other technologies and institutions. Artificial selection – agile, reflective and to some degree equipped with foresight – re-weaves the genetic and cultural legacy, only for this to be further re-woven in myriad struggles without any overall intent. The arts of civilisation, unless regularly renewed, are forever at risk of being overwhelmed by the wild, whether biotic or social.

In human affairs, the wild is shaped in particular by the powerful and the predatory. Fundamental choices of public policy and purpose are therefore posed, as to the directions of change that citizens and policy-makers wish to cultivate, modifying the interests and power that dominate the positional struggle. This is husbandry of the social fabric, applying the arts of civilisation to society as a whole. It is in these terms that we now examine public policy.

This brings us to a second answer to the question: 'What sort of policy science is implied by this evolutionary legacy?' It is an answer that is most obviously illustrated by reference to *social* policy. Maybe it is first necessary to consider what we mean by social policy. As an academic field, it lacks the simple clarity of the Walrasian tradition in economics. In terms of methods and paradigms, its exponents are rather promiscuous: as ready to deploy the legacy of Walras as that of Veblen. What they have in common, however – and perhaps this is all – is their concern *to analyse and evaluate the economy by reference to social goals such as equity and cohesion, defined politically for the society as a whole:* in other words, by reference to an overall normative and political intent. Already this challenges Walras, who presents the economy as an equilibrium which neither needs nor can admit any social challenge. However, it also challenges any evolutionary perspective on economy and society that imports from Darwin's account of natural selection the assumption of blind and unintended order or 'self-organisation'. It asserts instead that social progress is indeed possible: albeit progress defined within the particular historical circumstances of the academic and political actors concerned and therefore forever open to critical review and redefinition.

Social policy – as an academic discipline and as a form of political practice – applies the arts of civilisation to society as a whole. Just as the pigeon breeder or horticulturalist seeks to 'improve on nature' in regards to the latest generation of offspring and have it accord more fully with human purposes, social policy as political practice properly seeks to modify the positional struggles unfolding across economy and society, so that they accord more fully with whatever social goals the practitioner in question posits. Social policy as an academic discipline must equip political actors to reflect on those processes and civilise their consequences.

This then raises questions about economic policy also. We may of course conceive of economic policy as simply lubricating the Walrasian market, so that it can more readily attain its 'natural equilibrium'. Or in a watered-down form of Keynesianism, economic policy may be seen as simply managing the aggregate level of demand, so as to maintain full employment, leaving the market system otherwise to find its own equilibrium state. Or in the Schumpeterian tradition, economic policy-makers may be expected to stimulate entrepreneurial creativity and to guarantee property rights, but otherwise not to interfere in the economy's self-organising propensities (Parker and Stacey, 1994; Dopfer and Potts, 2008).

Against this, however, we may insist that economic policy, like social policy, is properly concerned with social goals such as equity and cohesion. Both social and economic policy – and indeed environmental and many other areas of public policy – are part of our endeavour to civilise the wild, bridling predation and barbarism. Even this however is not the end of the matter. Social policy may be part of our endeavour to civilise the wild; it is, however, still organised largely at the level of the nation state. It defines the institutional boundaries of citizenship,

46 Transformative realism

excluding outsiders or incorporating them on adverse terms. Moreover, by building loyalty and cooperation, risk sharing and collective action, it is an instrument in the positional struggle between nations, mobilising populations for economic and political competition (Titmuss, 1963; Room, 2004). This is as likely to fragment as to foster global civility. Whether, as a species, we are the capable of pooling the arts of civilisation, in a *globally* shared endeavour, remains to be demonstrated.

Notes

1 A previous version of this chapter appeared in the journal *Policy and Politics*: see Room (2012). I am grateful to the editor and publisher for permission to draw on that article.
2 This does not mean overlooking that human beings are biological organisms. They feed on other organisms; they are vulnerable to the ravages of new viruses; much of their economic and social activity is geared to the collective management of these challenges (Flannery, 1994: Part 2). Nevertheless, the variations that are thrown up in their social and economic technologies – and which are then variously selected and retained – are not biological. It is in this narrow sense that the analysis of societal evolution can, and should, ignore the biology.
3 Darwin was greatly influenced by Malthus, in describing the 'struggle for existence' that he saw in the wild, driving natural selection. The struggle for subsistence may similarly drive social interactions in the poorest human societies. More generally, however, it is hardly the case that entrepreneurs bestir themselves only when and if starvation threatens. Instead, it seems plausible to argue that it is the fear of loss of positional advantage and security that drives their incessant activity (Dopfer and Potts, 2008: para. 4.2.1).
4 Bronowski elaborates this theme more than Darwin does himself. Notice how this view of the self-creation of the human species also resonates with Marx's *Economic and Philosophic Manuscripts of 1844*, produced in the same year as Darwin's first draft of *Origin of Species* (and, like that, unpublished at the time). Little wonder that Marx and his followers have been keen to see themselves as fellow travellers with Darwin, in revealing in what human distinctiveness consists (Avineri, 1968: ch. 3; Schmidt, 1971: ch. 1).
5 We would be wrong to assume that anthropogenic change has become significant only in recent times. Flannery (1994) argues its major significance ever since the dawn of *Homo sapiens*.
6 Hodgson rejects the attempt by some scholars to substitute artificial for natural selection when applying Darwinian evolution to social and economic change (Hodgson, 2002; Hodgson and Knudsen, 2010: ch. 3). It might seem, therefore, that his critique applies here. Nevertheless, the present chapter is more nuanced, insisting that artificial and natural selection have to be understood by reference to their complex interrelationships.
7 It may be objected that rational action theory in at least some of its forms is far from 'timeless'. 'Rational expectations' theory, for example, is centrally concerned with future events. Nevertheless, the whole basis of rational expectations theory – as applied to financial markets for example – is that the probabilities of those future events can be calculated. Uncertainty (as distinct from risk) can therefore in principle be disregarded (Skidelsky, 2009: ch. 2).
8 This difference in ontology and focus goes wider than this of course. Thus, for example, debates over rational action and choice (including game theory) have given central attention to the conditions under which it may be rational for actors to cooperate or

even to behave altruistically (see, for example, Axelrod, 1984; Ball, 2004: chs 17–18). For us, it is certainly important to understand the conditions under which cooperation develops, rather than competition or conflict. Nevertheless, once we move from rational choices on relatively stable terrains to agile choices on turbulent terrains, it is the positional struggle that moves centre-stage. Competition and cooperation, solidaristic as distinct from individualistic advance, domination and adverse incorporation are contingent expressions of that struggle and must be understood in relation to it.
9 The classic discussion of contingency in evolution is Gould (1991: chs IV–V).
10 Meanwhile these mental models themselves evolve, in the sense that they are themselves subject to innovation and selective adaptation by the population of entrepreneurs. This is creativity as a collective cultural process; and here again there is path dependency. See, for example, Beinhocker's (2007: ch. 15) discussion of business plans.
11 This too is therefore an if-then search of the sort discussed earlier. If the arena chosen for selective probing offers scope for runaway advances, they are pursued; however, when such advance falls below some threshold level, the entrepreneur turns to other arenas, using the new leverage and vantage point gained.
12 Marris (1996: ch. 7) offers a similar account of power as 'the mastery of contingencies rather than the accumulation of assets'. He emphasises that at every level this typically involves the progressive displacement of the burden of uncertainty onto those who are weaker.
13 The theory of group-level or multi-level selection has in recent years become fashionable in evolutionary social science (Boyd and Richerson, 2002; Bowles, 2003; Sloan Wilson, 2008). The shift in vantage point adopted in this chapter, centred on artificial selection, also gives a key place to group selection: but in terms of the struggle for positional advantage through new lines of institutional differentiation in the population, consolidating some groups and incorporating others on adverse terms. Rather than blind population selection by reference to the 'fitness' of different groups, this is now a matter of differential power: a concept that has had little or no place within evolutionary social science, but is central once we 'reverse Darwin's journey'.

References

Abbott, A. (2001), *Time Matters: On Theory and Method*, Chicago, IL: University of Chicago Press
Akerlof, G.A. and P.M. Romer (1993), *Looting: The Economic Underworld of Bankruptcy for Profit*, Cambridge, MA: NBER Working Paper No. R1869 2
Arthur, W.B., S.N. Durlauf, and D.A. Lane (eds) (1997), *The Economy as an Evolving Complex System II*, Boulder, CO: Westview
Avineri, S. (1968), *The Social and Political Thought of Karl Marx*, Cambridge: Cambridge University Press
Axelrod, R. (1984), *The Evolution of Cooperation*, New York: Basic Books
Ball, P. (2004), *Critical Mass: How One Thing Leads to Another*, London: Heinemann
Beinhocker, E.D. (2007), *The Origin of Wealth*, London: Random House
Bowker, G.C. and S.L. Star (2002), *Sorting Things Out: Classification and Its Consequences*, Cambridge, MA: MIT Press
Bowles, S. (2003), 'The Co-evolution of Individual Behaviors and Social Institutions', *Journal of Theoretical Biology*, 223(2): 135–47
Boyd, R. and P.J. Richerson (2002), 'Group Beneficial Norms Can Spread Rapidly in a Structured Population', *Journal of Theoretical Biology*, 215(3): 287–96
Bronowski, J. (1981), *The Ascent of Man*, London: Futura
Brummer, A. (2009), *The Crunch: How Greed and Incompetence Sparked the Credit Crisis*, London: Random House

Coleman, J. (1990), *Foundations of Social Theory,* Cambridge, MA: Harvard University Press

Crouch, C. (2005), *Capitalist Diversity and Change: Recombinant Governance and Institutional Entrepreneurs,* Oxford: Oxford University Press

Darwin, C. (1859), *The Origin of Species,* London: Wordsworth (reprinted 1998)

Dawe, A. (1970), 'The Two Sociologies', *British Journal of Sociology,* 21(2): 207–18

Dawkins, R. (1976), *The Selfish Gene,* Oxford: Oxford University Press

Dopfer, K. and J. Potts (2008), *The General Theory of Economic Evolution,* London: Routledge

Douglas, M. (1986), *How Institutions Think,* London: Routledge and Kegan Paul

Flannery, T. (1994), *The Future Eaters,* New York: Grove Press

Galbraith, J.K. (2009), *The Predator State,* New York: Free Press

Gilbert, N. (2008), *Agent-Based Models,* London: Sage

Goldthorpe, J.H. (2000), *On Sociology,* Oxford: Oxford University Press

Goldthorpe, J.H. (2007), *On Sociology (2nd edition): Volume One: Critique and Program,* Stanford, CA: Stanford University Press

Gould, S.J. (1991), *Wonderful Life,* Harmondsworth: Penguin

Gould, S.J. and N. Eldridge (1977), 'Punctuated Equilibrium: The Tempo and Mode of Evolution Reconsidered', *Paleobiology,* 3: 45–51

Harré, R. (1972), *The Philosophies of Science,* Oxford: Oxford University Press

Hedström, P. (2005), *Dissecting the Social: On the Principles of Analytical Sociology,* Cambridge: Cambridge University Press

Hirsch, F. (1977), *Social Limits to Growth,* London: Routledge and Kegan Paul

Hodgson, G.M. (1998), 'On the Evolution of Thorstein Veblen's Evolutionary Economics', *Cambridge Journal of Economics,* 22: 415–31

Hodgson, G.M. (2002), 'Darwinism in Economics: From Analogy to Ontology', *Journal of Evolutionary Economics,* 12: 259–81

Hodgson, G.M. and T. Knudsen (2010), *Darwin's Conjecture: The Search for General Principles of Social and Economic Evolution,* Chicago, IL: University of Chicago Press

Kaldor, N. (1985), *Economics without Equilibrium,* Cardiff: University College Cardiff Press

Kauffman, S.A. (1993), *The Origins of Order: Self-Organisation and Selection in Evolution,* Oxford: Oxford University Press

Kellehear, A. (2007), *A Social History of Dying,* Cambridge: Cambridge University Press

Le Page, M. (2011), 'Unnatural Selection: How Humans are Driving Evolution', *New Scientist,* (2810) (27 April): 32–3

Loasby, B. (1999), *Knowledge, Institutions and Evolution in Economics,* London: Routledge

Marris, P. (1996), *The Politics of Uncertainty,* London: Routledge

Maynard Smith, J. and E. Szathmary (2000), *The Origins of Life: From the Birth of Life to the Origins of Language,* Oxford: Oxford University Press

Nelson, R. and S. Winter (1982), *An Evolutionary Theory of Economic Change,* Cambridge, MA: Harvard University Press

North, D.C. (1990), *Institutions, Institutional Change and Economic Performance,* Cambridge: Cambridge University Press

Odling-Smee, F.J., K.N. Laland, and M.W. Feldmann (2003), *Niche Construction,* Princeton, NJ: Princeton University Press

Parker, D. and R. Stacey (1994), *Chaos, Management and Economics: The Implications of Non-Linear Thinking,* London: Institute of Economic Affairs

Pierson, P. (2004), *Politics in Time,* Princeton, NJ: Princeton University Press
Pollan, M. (2003), *The Botany of Desire,* London: Bloomsbury
Pollan, M. (2006), *The Omnivore's Dilemma,* London: Bloomsbury
Potts, J. (2000), *The New Evolutionary Microeconomics: Complexity, Competence and Adaptive Behaviour,* Cheltenham: Edward Elgar
Room, G. (2004), 'Multi-Tiered International Welfare Systems', in I.R. Gough, G.D. Wood, A. Barrientos *et al.* (eds), *Insecurity and Welfare Regimes in Asia, Africa and Latin America,* Cambridge: Cambridge University Press: 287–311
Room, G. (2012), 'Evolution and the Arts of Civilisation', *Policy and Politics,* 40(4): 453–71
Schmidt, A. (1971), *The Concept of Nature in Marx,* London: New Left Books
Schumpeter, J.A. (1934), *The Theory of Economic Development,* Cambridge, MA Harvard University Press
Shubin, N. (2008), *Your Inner Fish,* Harmondsworth: Allen Lane
Skidelsky, R. (2009), *Keynes: The Return of the Master,* London: Allen Lane
Sloan Wilson, D. (2008), 'Multilevel Selection Theory and Major Evolutionary Transitions', *Current Directions in Psychological Science,* 17(1): 6–9
Soros, G. (2008), *The New Paradigm for Financial Markets,* London: Perseus Books
Streek, W. and K. Thelen (eds) (2005), *Beyond Continuity: Institutional Change in Advanced Political Economies,* Oxford: Oxford University Press
Tett, G. (2009), *Fool's Gold,* London: Little, Brown
Tily, G. (2007), *Keynes's General Theory, The Rate of Interest and 'Keynesian' Economics: Keynes Betrayed,* London: Palgrave Macmillan
Titmuss, R.M. (1963), 'War and Social Policy', in (ed.), *Essays on the Welfare State,* London: Unwin
Toner, P. (1999), *Main Currents in Cumulative Causation: The Dynamics of Growth and Development,* London: St Martin's Press
Veblen, T. (1898), 'Why is Economics not an Evolutionary Science?', *The Quarterly Journal of Economics,* 12(4): 373–97
Veblen, T. (1899), *The Theory of the Leisure Class,* New York: Macmillan
Weber, M. (1949), *The Methodology of the Social Sciences,* New York: Free Press

3 Contingent development and explanation

With Graham K. Brown

3.1 Introduction

Chapter 1 was concerned with complex systems and the non-linear dynamics they exhibit. However, as we noted there, much of the social world can be quite well described in linear terms: and social science offers a powerful array of technically sophisticated methods for modelling linear systems, in terms of independent and dependent variables.

The present chapter is concerned with the limits of such approaches and seeks to articulate a clear non-linear alternative: an alternative on which subsequent chapters can then draw. For that alternative it draws in particular on the evolutionary perspectives presented in Chapter 2. Evolutionary dynamics provide one of the principal examples of complex systems cited in the literature.

Here, as in Chapter 1, we do not reject linear models, but we do seek to establish their limitations and to develop a robust case for our alternative. As we shall see, the weaknesses we identify in linear models point directly towards the core strengths of this rival.

3.2 The General Linear Model

The task of social science is to explain social phenomena. This, it is commonly asserted, involves measuring the effects of different 'independent' variables on some 'dependent' variable of interest. This can be presented diagrammatically. In Figure 3.1, the independent variables x_1, x_2 and x_3 shape the dependent variable y, with some effects exerted via the intermediate variable z.

This vision or ontology of the social world can also be presented as a set of equations:

$$y = f_1(x_1) + f_2(x_2) + \ldots f_n(x_n) \tag{1}$$

This might be a single equation – or a whole set of equations that we solve simultaneously.

In order to isolate the separate causal effects of these independent variables, it is necessary to show that there are no significant interactions among them.

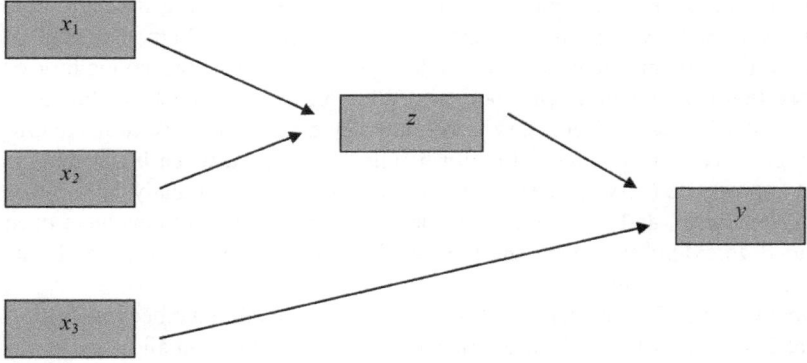

Figure 3.1 The General Linear Model

Much of the challenge of social science lies in deciding what to do when such interactions are present and substantial. Their presence can also, however, be used as a clue, to discover the underlying processes which may be at work.

Quantitative social science applies this vision using regression analysis. It casts the problem of explanation in terms of a set of linear equations: this is why it is often referred to as the 'General Linear Model' (GLM) (Abbott, 2001b: ch. 1). The GLM looks for the straight line (through n + 1 dimensional space) that best estimates – and therefore 'explains' – the dependent variable y as the additive outcome of a set of independent variables $x_1 \ldots x_n$ plus a random error term u:

$$y = b_1 \cdot x_1 + b_2 \cdot x_2 + \ldots b_n \cdot x_n + u \tag{2}$$

It is hardly surprising that the GLM exerts such a powerful sway across many disciplines. It is readily visualised; it can be formalised in terms of simple equations; it is convenient and tractable. It has admittedly been subject to criticism, questioning its general applicability to the real world. Even so, the linear model is often a useful first step in making sense of it (Jervis, 1997: 260–1).

3.3 Limitations of the GLM

The social world is not in general linear, but linear methods can often be used to good effect. However, this requires simplifying assumptions; and those assumptions must be defended. In this, the social sciences differ little from the natural sciences.

Among natural scientists, there are clear and well-recognised limits on applying linear models to particular phenomena. They assume, first, little or no interaction among the independent variables in question, so that their separate effects can be isolated and added. Second, they assume that changes in the independent variables will consistently produce proportional changes in the dependent variable. Neither of these assumptions holds generally: linear systems, therefore, are almost always understood to be 'local' approximations of non-linear systems. (In the language of Chapter 1, they are thus treated as though they were closed systems, having little or no interaction with the larger environment.) With this proviso, much can be done.

In social science, it is necessary to be similarly clear as to these limits and to have alternative strategies available, for handling problems, when linear models are not appropriate (Jervis, 1997: 34ff.). Using linear forms of analysis as a first step can be useful, and over recent decades smart technical solutions have been developed, to extend the scope and power of the GLM. Nevertheless, the limits discussed above are real.

In many areas of social science, linear analysis seems to have become a form of what Kuhn (1970) described as 'normal science', with anomalies and problems being 'explained away' or put on one side (Laitin, 2003; Stolzenberg, 2003). Nevertheless, a number of scholars have argued that these anomalies require a paradigmatic shift: or at least recognition that where linear methods are inappropriate, alternatives must be developed. It is to this task that this chapter will be devoted. We start with some of the concerns about the GLM which that critical scholarship has identified: concerns that echo the well-recognised limits we have just highlighted on the application of linear models.

Interacting variables and their separate effects

In some empirical situations, the independent variables interact with each other. Now the corresponding equations (such as equation (1) above) cannot in general be solved mathematically; and within statistical models (such as (2) above), these interactions will potentially produce bias in both estimators and significance for each of the variables in question.

Nevertheless, all is not lost. The stability and dynamics of such non-linear systems can be explored, including by computational methods. In terms of statistical models, it may to some degree be possible to deal with these problems through smart technical 'fixes'.[1] It can also be useful to ask just *why* these interactions are present and substantial: and to use them as a clue, to point to the deeper underlying variables or processes that may be at work. It is after all precisely by confronting inconsistencies in this way that scientific understanding and practice are able to advance (Kuhn, 1970; Popper, 1994: ch. 5; Tavory and Timmermans, 2014).

Thus, for example, Abbott studies interactions among variables in order to decide at what 'level' to study urban systems. He reviews studies of city neighbourhoods undertaken by the Chicago school of sociology in the inter-war period (Abbott, 1997). Some neighbourhoods had connections to the larger city that were limited and rather stable: their development could therefore be studied in terms of factors endogenous to the neighbourhood in question. Others, however, were involved in regular interactions with other neighbourhoods, which to some degree shaped their development. One community might thus find itself dancing to the rhythms of another. Finally, for some neighbourhoods these interactions across the city were so intense that it was necessary to focus attention not on individual communities, but on these larger processes, and on the cascades of change they unleashed across the city, albeit on a scale and to a timing that were not foreseeable. In this way, the interactions that Abbott observes – with their sudden and disproportionate effects – prompt us to rethink the social systems with which we are confronted and their dynamic connections.

It is true that when confronted, for example, with differences in rates of poverty or unemployment, across these city neighbourhoods, we can use multi-level modelling. This will allow us to disentangle the effects of differences in the characteristics of individuals living in different areas from the higher-level effects of differences between the areas (for example, in terms of their proximity to industrial regions). What such methods cannot do is unpick the interconnections of those neighbourhoods – the industrial ecologies within which employment is generated – and the path dependencies involved in their interrelated histories. An example of just such a study appears in Chapter 7 of this book, as Annex 7.2. This refers to the Community Development Project (CDP) launched by the UK government during the 1970s. It provides an analysis of the economic and industrial development of different neighbourhoods, driven predominantly by the economic interests of corporations and better-off communities within the city (CDP Inter-Project Editorial Team, 1977).

A further example is provided by Brown and Langer (2011). They review quantitative comparative studies of civil conflict. The chances of civil conflict across much of the developing world have been significantly reduced, compared with the period of the Cold War. Scholars have typically handled this by incorporating a Cold War 'dummy' variable into their explanatory equations. Brown and Langer, however, question this approach, unless the dummy can be given some theoretical or ontological significance. Instead, what the dummy reflects is a different global context: the reconfiguration of the international system, moving it away from a bipolar world. These global conditions, very different during and after the Cold War, affected the relations between the various factors within individual countries associated with civil conflict. The end of the Cold War constituted a 'structural break' in global context that changed not just the statistical significance but also the causal direction among some country-level variables.

In both of these examples – the neighbourhoods of Chicago and the war-torn countries of the developing world – any attempt to apply linear explanatory models is vitiated by connections with the larger world. GLM orthodoxy takes the system of equations as self-contained, within a closed system: all else is taken as given. Empirically, however, there are contextual contrasts that affect how these models play out. Moreover, any real-world system sits within a larger context, which is liable to shape the relationships between independent and dependent variables. In such cases, the GLM offers no universal truths: at best just truths that are context-dependent.

It is not just that the larger context may shape the relationships between the independent and dependent variables. As we saw in Chapter 1, open systems of this sort encounter positive and negative feedback from the larger environment in which they are embedded, and which they simultaneously reshape. These positive feedbacks drive them away from their starting position, in terms of the configurations ('self-organisation') that they take and the properties of the systems they generate.

Disproportional effects

The GLM assumes that changes in the independent variables will consistently produce proportional changes in the dependent variable across the entire range of observable values. It assumes moreover that these effects unfold within a very simple 'timescape'. The independent variables all act, all of the time, and the changes they produce in the dependent variable are within the same timescale.

In the empirical social world, timescapes are more complex. Some effects are short-term and immediate, while others are long-term and delayed (Abbott, 2001b: ch. 1). Many social processes are replete with time lags, ratchets and path dependencies (Lieberson, 1987: ch. 4). Pierson (2004: 74–7) points to the consequences of long-term and often slow changes in background social and economic conditions. The effects of this cumulative shift need not be gradual and continuous; there may, rather, be long periods of stasis, and then thresholds at which sudden avalanches of reconfiguration occur, sometimes discussed in terms of 'punctuated equilibria'.[2]

It is possible for the GLM to handle some of these temporal complexities using more sophisticated statistical techniques. Abbott's critics claim that he caricatures quantitative sociologists as naive researchers who 'have not heard about' advanced econometric techniques such as structural equation modelling (SEM), time series analysis and hierarchical linear models (Stolzenberg, 2003: 422). In the decade or so since the first publication of Abbott's critique, the rapid progress of computational power and statistical sophistication have reinforced this rejoinder.

Nevertheless, these temporal complexities, taken together, point to fundamental difficulties for the GLM, when applied to social sub-systems and processes with complex interconnections. It is these connections, short-range and long-range, that can produce disproportional change across complex timescapes, with apparent stasis in the short run hiding long-distance changes and long-term shifts.

What this also means is that change is not just non-proportional in a quantitative sense: it can also involve wholesale reconfiguration. Here are 'variables' that emerge, divide, amalgamate and disappear, and among which relationships develop and change. For understanding these dynamics, the techniques of the GLM are of little use.

Here again, therefore, these departures from the GLM provide us with clues about the deeper processes that are going on. Neither the natural nor the social world is linear: where linear methods can be used to good effect, it is as 'local' approximations of non-linear systems. This presupposes little or no interaction with the larger environment. Where those interactions are significant, an alternative approach is needed.

All of these limitations of the GLM resonate with the discussion of complex systems in Chapter 1 and the non-linear dynamics they exhibit. The GLM is predicated on a rather static view of the social world that cannot do justice to the dynamic interrelations among actors and institutions that we examined there. Whether this is a price we are ready to pay, for its technical sophistication, may vary between research problems as well as between researchers: but it is a question which can hardly be avoided.

3.4 The evolutionary alternative

The GLM finds its inspiration in classical physics. Evolutionary biology provides a quite different source of conceptual and methodological inspiration – albeit one that social scientists have interpreted and applied in a diversity of ways.[3]

The strengths of an evolutionary model align closely with the weaknesses of the GLM discussed in the previous section. It is, therefore, by reference to such a model that we now construct an alternative ontology and methodology for social science, at least in relation to those empirical applications where the GLM is inappropriate.

Evolution as contingent development

Darwin (1859) offered an account of evolution through natural selection. The scarcity of food relative to the available population provokes an unending Malthusian competition for life, a 'struggle for existence'. However, in each generation some offspring offer new 'variations' which enable them to thrive and reproduce with greater success within their particular environment. These superior varieties then become progressively better-represented in successive generations. It is from these blind population dynamics – 'blind' in that there is no overall intent or purpose – that the differentiation and adaptation of species arise.

In modern Darwinism, we understand biological variations in terms of genetic recombinations and mutations. Each generation of a population throws up new variations of its genetic legacy. It is upon these that natural selection operates within a given environment, allowing some of these variations to thrive more than others. Henceforth it is *their* genetic make-up that will be preponderant within the species concerned. The direction of such evolutionary development of a species is, however, by no means random. Its genetic legacy encodes past investments, enabling but also limiting and channelling subsequent development (Shubin, 2008). History matters: evolution is path-dependent.

An evolutionary journey can be visualised as an adaptive walk across a fitness landscape (Kauffman, 1993). No species makes its journey in isolation. The fitness landscapes of different species are linked. They co-evolve. In some cases this is an antagonistic process, an 'arms race' between predator and prey species. In others it is a process of mutually beneficial adjustment, as for example between insects and flowering plants. The evolutionary journey of a given species, re-weaving its genetic legacy and developing its potentialities, is path-dependent

56 *Transformative realism*

therefore by reference not only to that legacy, but also to the ecosystems of which it has become part. It is on the sequence-contingent combination of this dual legacy that natural selection acts.

The classic discussion of contingency in evolution is Gould (1991: chs IV–V). The various species alive today have evolved from common ancestors, as depicted in Darwin's famous 'Tree of Life', reproduced in Figure 3.2 (Darwin, 1859). What Gould challenges is the assumption that only a few branches of that tree have been extinguished along the way. Drawing on evidence of the explosion in new species during the Cambrian period, and the mass extinction of the Permian, Gould argues that many whole branches have disappeared: subsequent speciation has involved little more than additional twigs on the few branches that remained. More strongly, he argues that those species that failed to survive disappeared in brief episodes of mass extinction, involving exogenous shocks and cascades of eco-change. This is discontinuous change, in the form of 'punctuated equilibria', with periods of stasis followed by large-scale reconfiguration (Gould and Eldridge, 1977). Gould famously concludes that if the 'tape of history' were to be 'replayed' many times, altering some minor detail in that chain of contingencies, each would likely have produced a quite different result, few involving anything like *Homo sapiens*.

Flannery (1994) similarly unpicks the contingencies of the 'tape' of evolution in the lands of Australasia. In each case the co-evolutionary dynamics of the race for survival progressively transformed the environment in which natural selection acted. In New Zealand, birds came to dominate; in New Caledonia, reptiles; in Australia, marsupials. Flannery accounts for these contrasting

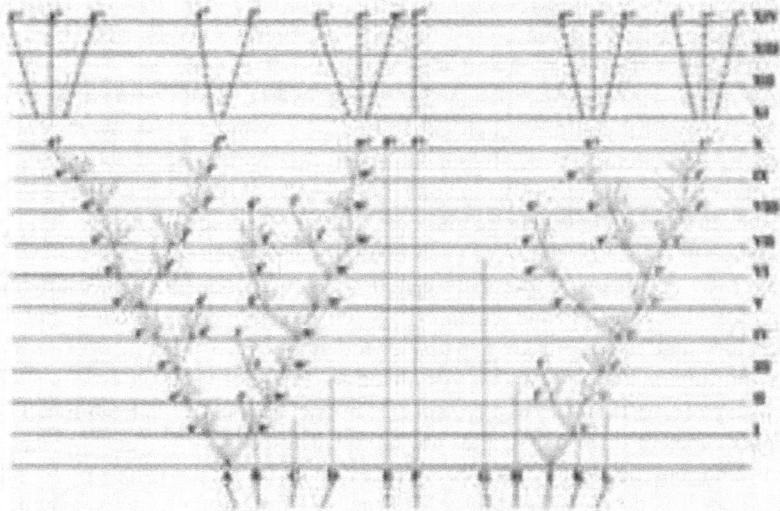

Figure 3.2 Darwin's Tree of Life

ecosystems by unpicking the successive connections and contingencies that this evolutionary history has entailed. He shows that the 'tape' can produce multiple 'narratives', albeit not without limit. Thus across these different ecosystems, Flannery identifies equivalent niches for particular birds, reptiles and marsupials, respectively, the counterparts of the major species of placental mammals on the Eurasian landmass. These are some of the limits on the tape of history, set by the interdependence of evolutionary niches (Solé and Bascompte, 2006: chs 4, 6).

Flannery turns finally to the arrival of humans: perhaps 60,000 years ago in Australia, 3,500 in New Caledonia, a mere 800 in New Zealand. The new predator initially enjoyed easy pickings. This initial plenty enabled rapid growth of the human population, but this led soon to ecological impoverishment. The human population of Australia eventually forged a new and sustainable niche for itself, long before Europeans arrived; in New Zealand in contrast, where there had been less time for such adjustment, it was a Hobbesian world of savage conflict that greeted the Europeans.

This was the major contingency that has shaped all these lands – the arrival of humans – not just the Europeans of recent times, but the Aboriginal peoples themselves. These, no less than the Europeans, were what Flannery terms the 'future eaters': a species that can readily shift the focus of its predations, even if the price paid is the spoliation of its own future. Here is no benign ecological 'balance' put at risk by the European incursion; no resilient Eden husbanded by ancient Aboriginal wisdom. Here, rather, is a story of environmental degradation and downward spiral (Flannery, 1994: ch. 21), albeit concealed from our eyes by its contingent complexity.

It is with just such complex and contingent processes of development that social as well as evolutionary science must grapple. This will, however, require that we include purposive human agency as well as 'blind' evolution. That is of course already present in Flannery's account, as he addresses the arrival of humans in Australasia, their social organisation and their predation. Before turning to those 'arts of civilisation' we consider how, in terms as abstract as our depiction of the GLM, we might capture the essential ingredients of evolutionary dynamics.

Modelling contingent development

With evolutionary science as our starting point, we now develop the 'Contingent Historical Model' (CHM), as an alternative to the GLM.

Figure 3.1 provided a visual representation of the GLM in its most basic terms. Such diagrams can provide powerful images that organise and direct our thinking about a given phenomenon. We now consider a corresponding representation of evolutionary dynamics, which in subsequent sections we can apply to the social world.

In his account of the diversification of species, Darwin was centrally concerned with processes of adaptation to the contingencies of different habitats. He depicted this visually as a 'Tree of Life', as reproduced in Figure 3.2

58 Transformative realism

(Darwin, 1859). This tree diagram offers successively sprouting branches and sub-branches, as particular 'variations' adapt to and exploit different habitats.

Here are just the sort of contextual contrasts with which our critique of GLM dealt, in the previous section. Real-world contexts vary: the explanations of real-world phenomena that we can expect to develop must be sensitive to these: truths are context-dependent. Causal analysis disentangles and peels away these contingencies. What the tree diagram does is set these contextual contrasts within a historical setting: a tree with a succession of ever-finer branches. When we come later to apply this to the social world, we will need to explain in social terms how the range of branches and choices is socio-structurally filtered and constrained (Abbott, 2001b: 250–8).

It is on ancestors and descendants that the image of the tree focuses our attention. Nevertheless, Darwin also referred to the *co-evolution* of species. His successors, even more, have shown how powerfully the dynamic synergies and arms races of co-evolution shape the evolutionary story (Kauffman, 1993; Maynard Smith and Szathmary, 2000). Such co-evolution typically involves populations that are far removed from each other in the evolutionary tree: for example, flowers and insects over the last 140 million years.

Think of looking down on the Tree of Life from above and viewing the top-most branches, the various species that are alive today: or indeed any other horizontal 'cut' representing the species that lived at another chosen period in the Earth's history. Across each of these cross-sections, the various branches (species) are connected in ecosystems of interdependence, which powerfully influence which of those species thrive and which are extinguished.

Consider Figure 3.3.

A and **B** (at the bottom of the diagram) are two mutually adapted entities in the world of today. They might, for example, be the populations of two species such as bees and flowering plants, benefitting each other's nourishment and reproduction.

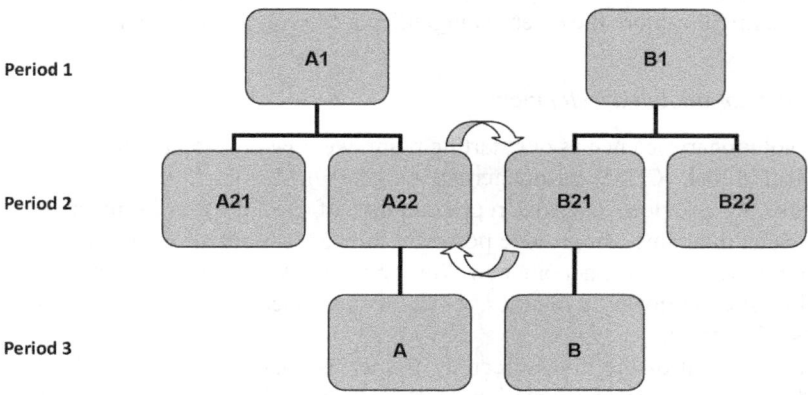

Figure 3.3 The Contingent Historical Model

We then pose the question: how did this mutual adaptation arise? We decline to treat it as a causal correlation, with the population of flowers 'causing' the population of bees within a timeless environment. Instead, we seek to unpick the intricate and messy history of successive contingencies that has led to the mutual adaptations of today.

The upper part of the diagram reveals those historical contingencies. **A1** and **B1** were the ancestors of today's bees and flowers. As we know from Darwin, in each generation, variations are produced. In general, however, as long as the environment remains stable (Period 1) they are unlikely to displace **A1** and **B1**.

It is when some environmental change occurs, at the start of Period 2, that we may expect some of the variations (**A21, A22, B21, B22**) to be adopted as superior to **A1** and **B1**, which now become extinct. However, which of the variations **A21** and **A22** becomes preponderant depends in part on the new biotic environment constituted by the arrival of **B21** and **B22**; and *vice versa*. In short, what is crucial is which of the four sets of interactions between **A21** and **A22** on the one hand, **B21** and **B22** on the other, is of greatest mutual benefit.

In the diagram, we show the relationship of **A22** with **B21** as being this favoured pairing, this synergy or 'elective affinity'.[4] Each will now accelerate the flourishing of the other. Their flourishing will in turn deny resources to **A21** and **B22**, which in the 'struggle for existence' become extinct. Hence we arrive at the bottom row of the diagram, Period 3, where **A** and **B** dominate. Here, by virtue of their domination, the environment is quite different from that in Period 1 or even in Period 2. And indeed, **A** and **B** are themselves quite different in their capacities from their respective forebears **A1** and **B1**: perhaps barely recognisable. Nevertheless, the domination of **A** and **B** is unlikely to last forever; further rounds of interaction with the wider ecosystem will eventually destabilise it, as new rounds of variation and selection are set in motion.

Most ecosystems are, of course, more complex than this, involving a larger number of species. Figure 3.3 is meant to capture this self-reinforcing process of mutual adaptation in its simplest, rather than its most typical form. That after all is the purpose of any canonical representation. Nevertheless, we briefly add a few further refinements.

First, we notice that local variations in environmental conditions can mean that an elective affinity that flourishes in one locality may be less successful in another. In some localities it may even be that **A21** and **B22** become the favoured pairing, gradually producing an ecology distinct from those where **A22** and **B21** dominate.

Second, we have seen that the 'elective affinity' between **A22** and **B21** accelerates the flourishing of both. In more complex ecosystems, this may then have consequences for other species **C**, **D** and **E**, with which they also interact. In some cases, those additional interactions may bring negative feedback, dampening and limiting the flourishing of **A** and **B**. In others, however, additional synergies may be uncovered, setting in motion more extensive cascades of reconfiguration across the ecosystem. Ecosystems are complex; their dynamics are contingent on these short- and long-range interactions; the specific outcomes are difficult to predict.

60 *Transformative realism*

The dynamic synergies between particular elements have as their obverse and their corollary the progressive disruption of other connections and elements of the ecosystem – and the incorporation of those elements into the 'empire' of the favoured elements (see Figure 3.4). The **A22–B21** axis becomes a vector of cumulative change around which the wider ecosystem is progressively reordered and reconfigured. This also makes it a non-linear system with strong path dependency, where instead of the additive effects that are central to the GLM, change is multiplicative and self-reinforcing.

The dynamic synergy cannot, however, continue without limit: nor can the concomitant destruction and recycling of other elements. Some parts of the wider ecosystem are too resilient and robust to be unpicked and reworked: they constitute an 'evolutionarily stable state' (Maynard Smith, 1982). Moreover, the cumulative change that is driven by the elective affinity of **A22–B21** is forever opening up new possibilities: even while **A22** and **B21** flourish more than ever before, new windows of opportunity have thereby been opened up for other elements of the ecosystem, other dynamic synergies that may eventually match or even surpass **A22–B21**.

3.5 The CHM and the arts of civilisation

The foregoing account of evolutionary dynamics resonates with our critique of GLM. It brings centre-stage systems of elements that interact with each other and with the larger environment. It encompasses complex 'timescapes', with path dependency and sudden but disproportionate effects. Here are 'variables' that emerge, divide, amalgamate and disappear, and among which relationships develop and change. Here, moreover, is acceptance – indeed insistence – that

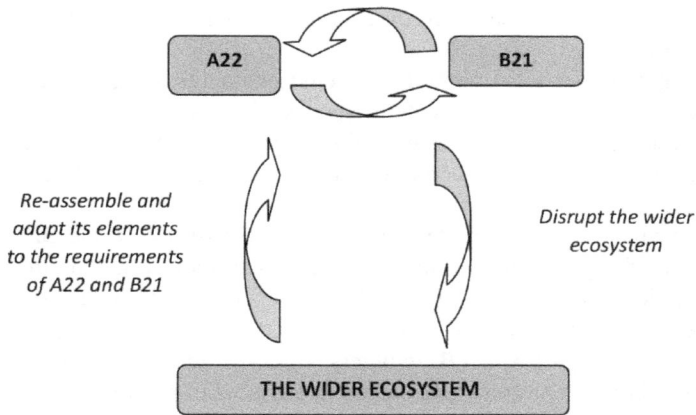

Figure 3.4 Creative destruction

change does not unfold within a stable environment, an unchanging given. For understanding these dynamics, the techniques of the GLM are of little use.

This evolutionary dynamic is the basis for our 'Contingent Historical Model'. The CHM thus rests on assumptions quite different from those of the GLM. It offers an evolutionary model of historical contingency which we will apply to the social world also: an alternative ontological and methodological inspiration. It is to the social world that we now turn.

The GLM involves a rather limited notion of social actors: they are little more than the arena within which the regression coefficients do their work. This is a perspective which sees individuals as simply adjusting to the changing social structures and circumstances in which they find themselves. In contrast, the CHM allows for a strong view of social action, which brings individual definitions of the situation centre-stage. Social systems now appear as the emergent outcome of social interactions among myriad individuals. If this outcome is orderly, it is so in part because some social actors have succeeded in negotiating or imposing that order on others. However, this is always provisional and contingent, in face of the ever-renewed struggle for positional advantage.

Evolution by natural selection is a blind process. In human societies, people to some degree make their own history. They probe and they experiment; they develop their understanding and their capacities. It is in these terms that we consider how human agents, by re-weaving their technological and institutional legacy, can probe and unlock the potentialities of their society and their world (see also Chapter 2 above). This is what earlier chapters referred to as the 'dance' between the self-organisation that may 'emerge' blindly at macro-level and the efforts of social actors to impose organisation and direction of their own.

The evolutionary journey again starts with novelty or variation: what we earlier described as diversification: referring now, however, not to genetic mutations, but to new combinations of the technological and institutional legacy. Among evolutionary economists, Potts (2000) adopts just such a combinatorial ontology, applied to technologies for purposes of production. A similar ontology is evident in Crouch (2005), applied to institutional innovations. Both writers highlight the role of entrepreneurs – whether in the realm of production or institutional governance – who rework these combinations, so as to better achieve their purposes (Room, 2011: ch. 6).

Human ingenuity here reworks the technological and institutional legacy, in hope of producing new variants more suited to human purposes (Potts, 2000; Beinhocker, 2007). Nevertheless, how a given technological innovation will fare – and how it may interact with other technologies and institutions – can never be entirely foreseen. Entrepreneurial ingenuity may *propose* new variants: but it is, these writers argue, processes of differential selection through the market that *dispose*; and these can be just as collectively 'blind' and devoid of overall intent as the processes of natural selection that drive speciation in the wild.

Even as those collectively blind processes unfold, however, strategically purposeful social actors will attempt to modify them to their own ends – depending on the resources and power at their disposal. Entrepreneurs are forever on the lookout for new co-evolutionary dynamics that will produce returns from relatively modest investments. Such dynamics may entail co-evolution between different technologies; between new technologies and new markets; between new forms of industrial organisation and new systems of public regulation, etc. To discover and nurture such dynamics is central to what we may call the arts of civilisation (Bronowski, 1981: chs 2–4).

This makes for non-linear change which is multiplicative and self-reinforcing, instead of the additive effects that are central to the GLM.[5]

3.6 Methodological implications

We now require an empirical methodology, appropriate to the dynamics of the CHM and applicable to the social world. In developing this methodology, we again take inspiration where appropriate from evolutionary biology, as well from social scientists who have sought to capture these dynamic processes in their empirical research.

At the heart of the CHM – and its parsimonious depiction in Figure 3.3 – is a dynamic ensemble of mutually adapted elements. This is an ensemble that has emerged from processes of mutual reinforcement: a process that crowds out or progressively dominates other elements. We seek an empirical methodology for analysing such dynamic ensembles in the social and political world and the processes of mutual adaptation from which they have emerged.

Qualitative system dynamics

Powell has developed qualitative system dynamics (QSD) for the analysis of institutional change: he builds on the work of such writers as Checkland and Coyle (Checkland and Scholes, 1990; Coyle, 1996; Powell and Bradford, 1998, 2000). He first maps the organisations of interest and the connections of interdependence they involve. He then labels each line of interdependence, to indicate its direction but also whether the relationship is direct or inverse: whether, in other words, an increase in some property or activity of the 'upstream' node causes a change in the 'downstream' node that is positive or negative.

Within this map, Powell proceeds to identify those cycles whose links are all positive. These are cycles which loop back on themselves in self-reinforcing circles. When any one element starts increasing, the whole sub-system experiences explosive growth; when any starts decreasing, the sub-system experiences implosive collapse. Powell refers to these as 'runaway loops'. In Figure 3.5 the runaway loop is marked as a dotted line. It is this loop, involving elements **A**, **B**, **F** and **C**, that is the counterpart to the elective affinity between **A22** and **B21** in Figure 3.3. Meanwhile other cycles of interdependence loop back on themselves, in ways that dampen down change and stabilise the system as it presently exists.

Runaway sub-systems such as these produce the processes of mutual reinforcement on which CHM centres. They enable particular ensembles of elements to

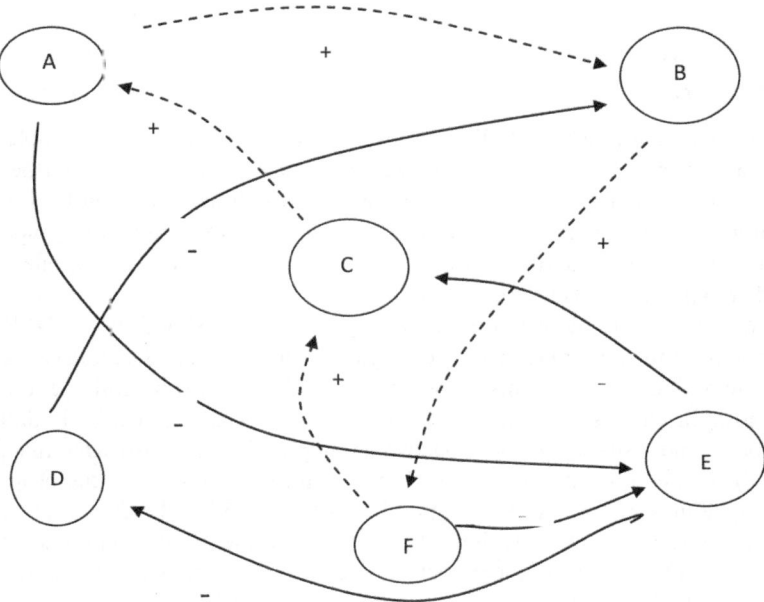

Figure 3.5 Runaway loops

form and flourish and eventually to dominate the system as a whole. Powell thus provides a useful step forward in our analytical quest.

Having identified the runaway loops, the next step is to assess how positive is positive: in other words, how strong is the self-reinforcing dynamic. This will determine the speed at which the cycle 'runs away'. Second, we need to know how well-connected is the sub-system or loop in question to the system as a whole, so that its runaway loops have wider influence. There may be particular threshold effects: beyond a certain point, the runaway sub-system triggers other sub-systems, which in their turn begin also to 'run away'. The particular dynamics that emerge will be heavily dependent on the way that elements are connected to each other.

Room shows how this approach can be applied in empirical research. He uses Powell's analysis of 'runaway loops' to examine the dynamics of secondary school choice in the UK and the processes of social class segregation which it tends to produce (Room, 2011: section 15.2). This he sets within the particular policy setting of competitive 'quasi-markets' that was introduced by the Conservative government and continued by New Labour after 1997.

Nevertheless, Powell's QSD assumes that the configuration of elements – in Figure 3.5, for example – remains fixed. There are no novelties and no extinctions. He does not allow for the sub-system that runs away to change its configuration or to reshape the larger system in which it is embedded. Powell advances our

64 *Transformative realism*

quest: but he does not provide us with a full analytic of CHM and its evolutionary ontology.

Autocatalytic sets

Like Powell, Jain and Krishna (2003) employ a methodology of directed graphs (networks where the *direction* of the connection matters).[6] They take us further than Powell, however, inasmuch as they investigate how 'runaways' can lead to the reconfiguration of particular sub-systems or, indeed, of the network or graph as a whole. Such reconfigurations are of course important to any evolutionary framework and therefore also for our CHM.

Jain and Krishna are interested in autocatalytic sets (ACS) and the key role that these appear to have played in the origins of life. An ACS comprises a set of simple molecular organisms, none able individually to self-replicate, but each providing a catalyst for each of its fellows: a process of symbiotic and co-evolutionary 'boot-strapping' for collective self-replication (see also Kauffman, 1993: ch. 7). Jain and Krishna use network or graph theory to explore the properties and dynamics of such ACSs, with a view to illuminating the dynamics of co-evolution more generally. It is these ACSs that form the close counterpart to Powell's treatment of runaway loops, but in an evolutionary setting, as required by our account of elective affinities and mutual adaptation (Figure 3.3).

As we have seen, Powell is particularly interested in sub-systems where all the links are positive. These are 'runaway' loops of mutual reinforcement and flourishing. Jain and Krishna incorporate these into their own analytical scheme, by modelling a population located at each of the different nodes, which then enjoys particularly rapid growth if it is part of an ACS (Section 3.3). Up to this point however, the analysis by Jain and Krishna – like that of Powell – does not allow for any reconfiguration of the system or any transformation of its elements.

Finally, however, they allow the network or graph itself to evolve, consistent with what happens in Darwinian evolution (Sections 3.4–3.5). It is those nodes whose populations are flourishing that are differentially retained – and, of course, these tend to be the ones favoured by ACSs. The least flourishing are extinguished. Random new nodes and connections are then added, mimicking the random mutations in Darwin. This is an evolving system, driven by the mutual reinforcement of the ACSs: no longer, therefore, does it have a fixed configuration, as in Powell's work. (For an example of one moment in this transformation, see Figure 3.6.)

Think again of the Tree of Life (Figure 3.2). Looking down from above and viewing the top-most branches, we see the various species that are alive today. Any other horizontal 'cut' will show the species that lived at another chosen period in the Earth's history. Across each of these cross-sections, the various branches (species) are connected in ecosystems of interdependence. It is with these horizontal cuts that Jain and Krishna are concerned.

The dynamic ensembles they model lie at the heart of the CHM. This is what we have presented as Figures 3.3 and 3.6. This must still however be used

(h) n = 6062

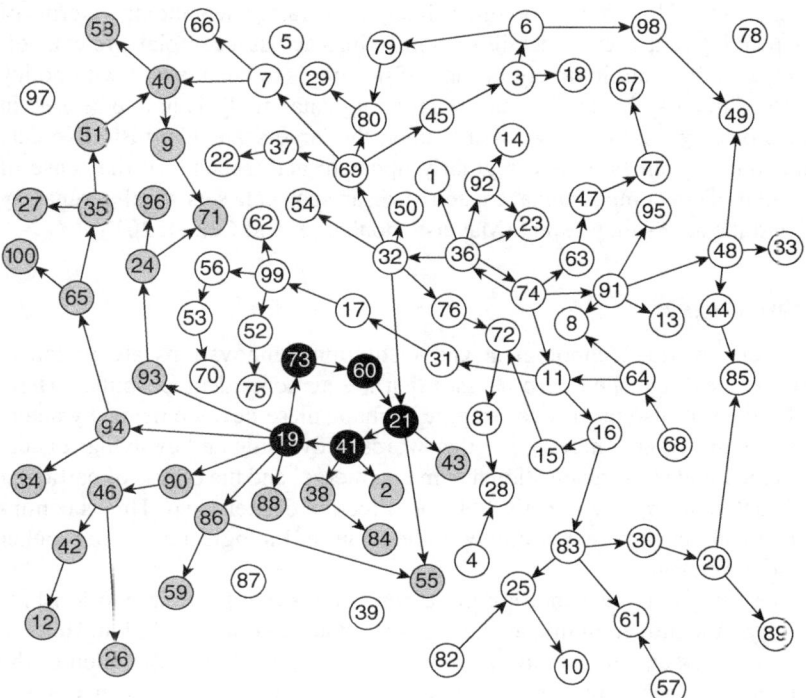

Figure 3.6 Jain and Krishna's autocatalytic sets

Source: Figure 3.6 is part of a diagram in Jain, S. and S. Krishna (2003), 'Graph Theory and the Evolution of Autocatalytic Networks', in S. Bornholdt and H.G. Schuster (eds), *Handbook of Graphs and Networks*, Weinheim: Wiley-VCH: 355–395. Reproduced with kind permission of Wiley publishers.

Note: Black nodes belong to the core of the dominant autocatalytic set of the graph, grey nodes to its periphery, and white nodes are outside the dominant autocatalytic set. This diagram shows run 6062 in the computational modelling of the graph (Jain and Krishna, 2003).

in conjunction with Figure 3.2. Depending on the ensembles that triumph in Figures 3.3 and 3.6, some branches of the Tree of Life will flourish, while others will be extinguished. Figure 3.2 thus records the successive triumphs and tragedies of the dynamic interactions unfolding within Figures 3.3 and 3.6. More than this, it defines the cast of actors who will now take part in future rounds of co-evolutionary interaction – future versions of Figures 3.3 and 3.6 – and it bequeaths them an ecosystem which they will then in turn re-weave.

This is the formal analytic that seems best to capture the dynamic processes of mutual adaptation at the heart of the CHM. It can be used in two complementary ways. First, Jain and Krishna use computational models to simulate what can happen in such a dynamic system, depending on the parameters and algorithms adopted. Second, computational models of this sort can then serve as ideal types, illuminating the range of dynamics to be found in the real world (Gilbert and Troitzsch, 2005). However, to do this is likely to be rather demanding in terms of data, depending as it does on details of connections across a complex system, collected repeatedly – and in timely fashion, if the aim is to engage also with policy audiences. This may be an obvious area for 'big data' analysis in two senses: in the sense of drawing as far as possible upon the large-scale administrative data that are routinely amassed and regularly updated; and, second, in the sense of deploying modern computational capacity to scan such data sets, for the 'runaway loops' and the ACSs they reveal (Mayer-Schonberger and Cukier, 2013).[7]

Purposive struggles

In the social world, technological and institutional innovations are variously picked up or extinguished by processes that are, to some degree, 'blind'. Here, however, there is also purposive struggle to shape these developments, by actors in positions of power. There is, in other words, a dynamic and evolving 'dance' between the blind self-organisation that may 'emerge' and the efforts of particular strategic actors to impose organisation and direction of their own. This is contingent historical development, not now in the realm of biological evolution, rather that of social change.

We need methods for capturing these purposive struggles. Jain and Krishna, in their dynamic model, mimicked natural selection and blind evolution. Here, in contrast, we seek also to capture *artificial* selection (recall our discussion of the relationship between natural and artificial selection in Chapter 2 of this book). This will involve purposive changes to the nodes and connections of the network, having regard to the ACSs that the various actors want to flourish. It will allow for alternative visions by competing protagonists and a struggle between them to shape the dynamics of change.

Koenig and his colleagues (Koenig *et al.*, 2008) model innovation networks in ways that build closely on Jain and Krishna. Here, however, the focus is not upon biological ecosystems but upon firms, the knowledge transfer that takes place between them and the learning-by-doing that this allows.[8] Koenig, like Jain and Krishna, explores the blind evolutionary dynamics of such a system: however, he also models individual firms making their own choices of connections by reference to a utility function. In short, he begins to model the arts of civilisation, though still only at the micro-level. Here are no large corporations – still less governments – making more extensive interventions in the 'ecosystem' and seeking to steer development in their own preferred direction.[9]

Notice that the network models offered by Jain and Krishna and by Koenig abstract from any differences in scale among the various players: the focus is entirely upon their elective affinities and the autocatalytic dynamics that these may engender. This ignores the hierarchical relationships of domination, protection and dependence, which are highly significant not only for human societies, but also within the food chains of the ecosystems with which evolutionary biologists are concerned (Solé and Bascompte, 2006). Again, however, all models and ideal types involve fateful choices as to what will be included: what is important is to draw all possible value from such models but also to recognise their limitations. Later chapters will give plenty of attention to the dynamics of such relationships between bigger and smaller actors.

Alongside this formal modelling, it may also be useful to use 'thick' qualitative and historical accounts. Given the evolutionary inspiration for our CHM, scholars who offer accounts of how institutions evolve would seem an obvious starting point. Thelen has been prominent among these (Thelen, 2004; Streek and Thelen, 2005). She and her collaborators provide examples of co-evolutionary dynamics that resonate with our own account of elective affinities and dynamic synergies. It is, for example, in precisely these terms that Palier investigates the 'Bismarckian' welfare states and their reforms during the last decade: how each reform impinges upon other elements of the welfare mix and, beyond that, upon employment structures and relations (Palier and Martin, 2008: ch. 1; Palier, 2010). He thereby makes sense of the sequence of actions by which policy-makers have set new dynamics in motion, undermining interests in the existing welfare settlement and building coalitions in support of change.

Meanwhile Esping-Andersen (1990) has spawned an influential stream of scholarship on the configurations into which national welfare systems fall. Using standard methods of correlation analysis, he maps the forms of stratification and political order mediated through welfare systems in different OECD countries and shows how these cluster into three principal regimes. He accompanies these comparative metrics with historical analysis. This is a story of social actors – in particular social classes – in a positional struggle on a landscape which is itself reshaped by that struggle. The latter involves the contested development of elective affinities between social actors and welfare terrains. Depending on the synergies that form, the welfare outcome tends to lock into one or other of Esping-Andersen's three regimes. Esping-Andersen is part of a larger literature, ranging across a variety of scientific disciplines, dealing with 'critical transitions' that may move social or physical systems between different 'regimes' (Scheffer, 2009).

Like Thelen, Esping-Andersen thus sits quite well within the CHM. This scholarship brings institutional contingency and evolution centre-stage. In both cases the starting point for the analysis is provided by various typical ensembles of associated elements in a state of mutual adjustment, interpreted as resulting from a history of successive contingent connections. Nevertheless, neither Esping-Andersen nor Thelen offers any formal models or tools that can bring analytical leverage to this history, allowing them to confirm, beyond the limited range of countries they study, the processes of evolution and lock-in that they infer.

The methodological programme and empirical research inspired and implied by the CHM might best use these two elements in combination: on the one hand, these 'thick' qualitative and historical accounts, on the other, the formal analytic displayed most parsimoniously by Figure 3.3 and given methodological content by Powell and by Jain and Krishna. Critics of the GLM have hitherto failed to develop an alternative which can match its attractions: its ease of visualisation, its formalisation in terms of simple equations, its convenience and tractability. They have therefore had an uphill task. The CHM as developed here shows what can be done.[10]

3.7 Conclusion

The limitations of the GLM need not mean its wholesale rejection. It is a matter of practical judgement how far it can still provide useful guidance for the analysis of particular empirical problems. The multiple contingencies of Figure 3.2, the transformative synergies of Figure 3.3, are not all-pervasive. Some degree of uniformity, stability and linearity remains (Jervis, 1997: 260–1). Figure 3.1 will often therefore remain a valuable point of reference.

The GLM and the CHM involve different notions of causation. The GLM aims to explain the quantitative value of the dependent variable y by reference to the independent variables $x_1 \ldots x_n$ as they act upon it. The variables themselves and their boundaries are fixed, as indeed are the relationships between them. Figure 3.1 presented the causal direction, from left to right, as the independent variables tightly influence the value of the dependent variable. Just how tight, depends on the proportion of variation in y for which we can thereby account: we may want to set some threshold for this proportion, before we can be satisfied with the causal explanation we have developed.

The practitioner of GLM searches for a system of independent variables whose effects on the dependent variable can be treated as a matter of linear addition. Indeed, much of the energy of the statistical community has been devoted to finding clever ways of doing this, even under apparently unpropitious circumstances. For CHM in contrast, we admit of a quite different class of phenomena: those whose configuration and frequency are driven by an interactive dynamic that is multiplicative not additive. This dynamic should not be seen as an inconvenience which the analyst must surmount or by-pass, but one which requires new and no less clever approaches. Here it is the 'elective affinities' among particular elements that lead to their progressive domination of the system in question and which CHM brings centre-stage. Figures 3.2 and 3.3 display complementary aspects of this causal dynamic.

In Chapter 1 we touched on generative mechanisms and causal powers, as discussed by realist writers such as Harré, in relation to both natural and social science (Harré, 1972; Harré and Secord, 1972: ch. 4). It is not enough to demonstrate, as GLM advocates, that the independent variables $x_1 \ldots x_n$ are statistically significant in determining the value of y: what is also necessary is to understand what generative capacities have been activated, to produce those effects, and what particular circumstances permitted this. The analysis of generative mechanisms aims at revealing such powers and contingencies. It is the interactive dynamic among populations of different species that provides the generative mechanism in Darwinian evolution: and that CHM inherits.

In human affairs these interactions are constructed institutionally and historically. If they are complex and contingent, subject to cascades of reconfiguration, this is because they are forever being contested and reshaped in the struggle for positional advantage. Harré's account of potentialities, critical thresholds and novel dynamics, can be read as much as an account of this historical and political struggle as a contribution to the philosophy of science.

This is contingent historical development, not in the realm of biological evolution, but rather in that of social change. It involves a struggle for positional advantage, which brings interests, power and politics centre-stage. In Chapter 1 we therefore referred to this perspective not as *evolutionary* but as *transformative realism*.

Nevertheless, two caveats are in order. First, it is necessary to avoid focusing attention only on the victors – the beneficiaries of the runaway cycles of mutual adaptation to which the CHM directs our attention. No less attention must be lavished on those elements and connections that are extinguished or, at least, subordinated and marginalised. This means unpicking the messy history of successive contingencies from which – had an alternative sequence of interactions occurred – a quite different dynamic of runaway and extinction would likely have emerged. This is central to Figure 3.3, concerned with synergies which on the one hand produce runaway flourishing, but on the other, domination and extinction.

Analysis guided by the CHM will start from an ensemble of mutually adapted elements and will then work back through the processes of mutual adaptation through which that ensemble emerged. However, it will also work forward from those origins, running alternative versions of Gould's 'tape of history' – alternative counterfactuals – for example, by comparative studies of the evolution of different welfare systems. In all of this, judgements of explanatory relevance will be needed, in selecting how far back to go, what institutional contexts to treat as significant, what range of comparisons to venture. The fruit of such enquiry is not the 'universal truths' about the causes of particular social outcomes to which the GLM aspires (albeit in the form of probabilistic statements), but 'time-bounded truths' about the contingent dynamics of social change (Brown and Langer, 2011).

There is a second caution. Even if we admit that social (like biological) development is captured more appropriately by CHM than by GLM, how fine-grained should our appreciation of historical contingency be? A variety of historical routes may lead to broadly the same destination; to delineate this variety may be of less importance than to explain how this single destination dominates them all. This is what von Bertalanffy (1968), one of the founders of the 'complexity' literature, refers to as the 'equifinality' of system trajectories towards particular 'attractor basins'.

The problem lies in knowing what individual detail can be neglected. This is, in one sense, a matter of being clear as to the theoretical – in this case sociological – questions that can sensibly be posed. It is also, however, a matter of being alert to the new elective affinities that may develop around some of those individual details. We need to be alert, not least because human actors are thus alert: on the lookout for opportunities to reshape their environment and to secure leverage for positional improvement. This probing and experimenting may then, for better or ill, set in motion larger-scale transformations. The future is always, to some degree, open.

Finally, the contrast between the GLM and CHM carries implications for how we understand the social sciences and the illumination they offer for policy-makers and public debate. The researcher must decide which of these two paradigms is appropriate in specific cases. This is not just a technical question. It involves judgements as to the significance of different dynamic synergies, in relation to the objectives not only of policy-makers, but also of other stakeholders across the communities affected. It is as we understand the historical contingencies that underlie the regularities and patterns of the world in which we live – and understand them by reference to the interests and power struggles involved – that we are better able to identify the policy choices and trade-offs that we confront (Jacobs, 2011).

Research for policy-making is a contested process, unavoidably involving interests and power and politics. Intrinsic to such struggles is the very definition of different societal 'problems'. Who is to be held accountable for these problems and what is the responsibility of the public authorities to address them? What standards of evidence are demanded for different problems, as a precondition for the investment of public resources? Which problems require a novel response – and when is such novelty no more than a way to avoid hard political questions?

For many exponents of GLM, the analysis of policy options and implications involves little more than the assessment of the regression coefficients: these are the 'drivers' of change which policy-makers must target (see, for example, Social Exclusion Unit, 2004). Nevertheless, it is common for a more complex array of causal processes – and therefore also policy levers – to operate. Lieberson (1987: ch. 5) questions the readiness of researchers to take the regression coefficients that emerge from such analysis as 'speaking for themselves' and revealing, on the basis of the variance they explain, the importance of different explanatory variables. He alerts us to the contingent and labile nature of these causal connections and the cascades of larger reconfiguration to which they may be subject, as a result of policy interventions that may have a narrower and more specific focus (chs 4, 11).

To what extent, therefore, can the CHM – suitably modelled and applied to empirical data – provide robust policy indicators and guidelines for a non-linear world? It is to this question that subsequent chapters of this book are in substantial part addressed.

Notes

1 If, for example, there is thought to be an interaction in the influence of two variables x_1 and x_2, we may create a third variable x_3, usually defined as the product of x_1 and x_2, which is then included in the regression analysis. Once this interaction term has been created, it allows us to maintain linearity in the estimation, if we assume that its influence is proportional to x_3. However, a limitation of this approach is that we need to stipulate *ex ante* what form the interaction takes.
2 Pierson (2004) notes that the current focus on short-term and immediate causes and effects was not always so: he cites the modernisation literature (p. 98), and its collapse in light of the critique that it faced, in terms of functionalism and teleology.

3 For an eloquent statement of the relevance of evolutionary models in social science, closely consistent with the argument of the present chapter, see Lieberson and Lynn (2002). See also Hodgson (2001: ch. 22; 2002) and Blaug et al. (2011). Contrast this with those who retain a focus on the biological substrate of human behaviour (for example, Sloan Wilson (2008)).
4 The term 'elective affinity' was originally used in German chemistry of the eighteenth century, to refer to the way in which compounds interact and combine selectively with each other (Howe, 1978). Goethe took this idea into his novel *Die Wahlverwandtschaften*, applying it to sexual attraction. Kant, in turn, applied the idea to relationships among concepts; Weber to relationships between ideas and the interests of social actors. Perhaps surprisingly, however, it does not seem to have been used in relation to biological co-evolution.

In these various cases, 'elective affinity' is not just a matter of complementarity or similarity: it is a dynamic synergy, in which elements that are especially favourable to each other enable the ensemble as a whole to flourish. In short, therefore, it offers a dynamic of mutual reinforcement and change. It is perhaps worth adding that the original search in German chemistry for such affinities was conducted in the shadow of Newton and in envy of physics and its claim to universal natural laws: just as our own account of CHM has been located within the larger debate about social science and that same Newtonian legacy of the GLM.
5 Other social scientists have similarly set such contingent variations within a historical setting: whether of individual social actors or of whole nations. Abbott (2001b: ch. 8), for example, thinks of social actors and their life histories as a succession of choices at 'turning points': transitions which will, he anticipates (p. 250), be revealed by the changed significance or polarity of country-level variables, in national trajectories before and after the transition.
6 Also available at http://arxiv.org/PS_cache/nlin/pdf/0210/0210070 v1.pdf
7 Goldthorpe (2007: ch. 6) proposes a marriage of rational action theory and large data sets: here in contrast we propose a marriage of transformative realism and big data.
8 This is very much in the tradition of economics writing on 'cumulative causation' including in particular Kaldor (Toner, 1999). It contrasts markedly with orthodox economics and its preoccupation with market 'equilibrium' (Kaldor, 1972). Also relevant here is the literature on national innovation systems (Lundvall et al., 2006).
9 One of my PhD students, Qin Zhang, based in Chongqing, China, has been using this framework to analyse the formation of industrial clusters. She explores how the city government, and multinational firms with a base in Chongqing, struggle to drive these location dynamics in different directions.
10 The methods we are advocating have affinities with some other theoretical toolkits. One good example is the approach to social movements and 'contentious politics' developed by McAdam, Tarrow and Tilly (2001). They shift the analysis of social mobilisation from 'static' and 'single actor' accounts to one focused on dynamic interactions, analogous to our shift from GLM to CHM. They analyse struggle in relation to the 'political opportunity structure', arguing that it is often *changes* in that structure that allow for major positional challenges. This is analogous to the introduction of a new 'species' into the Jain and Krishna system, prompting the emergence of a new autocatalytic set of previously lacklustre performers. Context and contingency, however, remain important in their account, as they do in the CHM. Thus in their comparative discussion of the dynamics of revolutionary mobilisation, country-specific cultural factors, and events such as the storming of the Bastille, retain an importance excluded from many more structural accounts of revolution such as those of Skocpol (1979).

Some writers on complexity, concerned with the same challenges as those discussed here, look to Ragin's Qualitative Comparative Analysis (QCA) as providing the way forward (Ragin, 1987: ch. 2). The GLM separates out the effects of individual causal variables on the dependent variable of interest. Ragin, in contrast, stresses that causal processes in social science typically involve multiple elements acting together. It is the intersection or conjunction of these elements that is necessary for a given causal process to operate.

Faced with an array of cases that involve combinations of these elements, Ragin asks which configurations give rise to the particular outcome of interest. For this purpose he uses Boolean algebra. This involves analysing cases by which elements are present or absent and recording whether, for the case in question, the outcome of interest is similarly present or absent. Elements and outcomes are thus forced into a simple either/or logic, displayed in a 'truth table' across the full range of the cases in question. (This approach in terms of 'crisp sets' has subsequently been modified by Ragin (2000), in the form of 'fuzzy' sets which can have intermediate values between zero and one, present and absent. For our present purposes however this modification is of marginal significance.)

This can, it might seem, be readily harnessed to the CHM. After all, Figure 3.3 took as its point of departure the ensemble of associated elements **A** and **B** in a state of mutual adjustment, the result of a history of successive contingent connections. However, CHM was concerned not only with the presence or absence of particular elements from a given ensemble, but also with the changing relations or connections among them. Truth tables ignore this (Crouch, 2005: 60) and the Boolean algebra says nothing about temporal processes (Abbott, 2001a). QCA can dissect what presently exists; it does not, however, shed light on the contingencies of yesterday, out of which this present has developed; nor does it encompass the further rounds of interaction and mutual adaptation that are liable to produce the elective affinities of tomorrow. Certainly QCA shows what co-presences of elements there are, but whether these have resulted from the successive mutual adaptations of the CHM, or have yet to undergo that mutually selective journey, is ignored.

Ragin has in recent years moved from QCA to the more general study of case studies, viewed as complex systems of interconnected elements (Byrne, 2005; Byrne and Ragin, 2009). This work, in conjunction with Byrne, claims inspiration from the 'complexity' literature that has emerged over recent decades. Whether these efforts will converge with our own account of CHM remains to be seen.

References

Abbott, A. (1997), 'Of Time and Space: The Contemporary Relevance of the Chicago School', *Social Forces*, 75(4): 1149–82

Abbott, A. (2001a), 'Review: "Fuzzy Set Social Science" by Charles Ragin', *Contemporary Sociology*, 30(4): 330–1

Abbott, A. (2001b), *Time Matters: On Theory and Method*, Chicago, IL: University of Chicago Press

Beinhocker, E.D. (2007), *The Origin of Wealth*, London: Random House

Blaug, M., G.M. Hodgson, O. Lewis, and S. Steinmo (2011), 'Introduction to the Special Issue on the Evolution of Institutions', *Journal of Institutional Economics*, 7(3): 299–315

Bronowski, J. (1981), *The Ascent of Man*, London: Futura

Brown, G. and A. Langer (2011), 'Riding the Ever-Rolling Stream: Time and the Ontology of Violent Conflict', *World Development*, 39(2): 188–98

Byrne, D. (2005), 'Complexity, Configurations and Cases', *Theory, Culture and Society*, 22(5): 95–111

Byrne, D. and C. Ragin (eds) (2009), *The Sage Handbook of Case-Based Methods*, London: Sage

CDP Inter-Project Editorial Team (1977), *The Costs of Industrial Change*, London: CDP Inter-Project Editorial Team

Checkland, P. and J. Scholes (1990), *Soft Systems Methodology in Action*, Chichester: John Wiley
Coyle, R. (1996), *Systems Dynamics Modelling: A Practical Approach*, London: Chapman and Hall
Crouch, C. (2005), *Capitalist Diversity and Change: Recombinant Governance and Institutional Entrepreneurs*, Oxford: Oxford University Press
Darwin, C. (1859), *The Origin of Species*, London: Wordsworth (reprinted 1998)
Esping-Andersen, G. (1990), *The Three Worlds of Welfare Capitalism*, Cambridge: Polity Press
Flannery, T. (1994), *The Future Eaters*, New York: Grove Press
Gilbert, N. and K.G. Troitzsch (2005), *Simulation for the Social Scientist (2nd Edition)*, Maidenhead: Open University Press
Goldthorpe, J.H. (2007), *On Sociology (2nd edition): Volume One: Critique and Program*, Stanford, CA: Stanford University Press
Gould, S.J. (1991), *Wonderful Life*, Harmondsworth: Penguin
Gould, S.J. and N. Eldridge (1977), 'Punctuated Equilibrium: The Tempo and Mode of Evolution Reconsidered', *Paleobiology*, 3: 45–51
Harré, R. (1972), *The Philosophies of Science*, Oxford: Oxford University Press
Harré, R. and P.F. Secord (1972), *The Explanation of Social Behaviour*, Oxford: Blackwell
Hodgson, G.M. (2001), *How Economics Forgot History*, London: Routledge
Hodgson, G.M. (2002), 'Darwinism in Economics: From Analogy to Ontology', *Journal of Evolutionary Economics*, 12: 259–81
Howe, R.H. (1978), 'Max Weber's Elective Affinities: Sociology within the Bounds of Pure Reason', *American Journal of Sociology*, 84(2): 366–85
Jacobs, A. (2011), *Governing for the Long Term*, Cambridge: Cambridge University Press
Jain, S. and S. Krishna (2003), 'Graph Theory and the Evolution of Autocatalytic Networks', in S. Bornholdt and H.G. Schuster (eds), *Handbook of Graphs and Networks*, Weinheim: Wiley-VCH: 355–95
Jervis, R. (1997), *System Effects: Complexity in Political and Social Life*, Princeton, NJ: Princeton University Press
Kaldor, N. (1972), 'The Irrelevance of Equilibrium Economics', *The Economic Journal*, 82(328): 1237–55
Kauffman, S.A. (1993), *The Origins of Order: Self-Organisation and Selection in Evolution*, Oxford: Oxford University Press
Koenig, M.D., S. Battiston, and F. Schweitzer (2008), 'Modeling Evolving Innovation Networks', in A. Pyka and A. Scharnhost (eds), *Innovation Networks: New Approaches in Modeling and Analyzing*, Heidelberg: Springer: 189–269
Kuhn, T.S. (1970), *The Structure of Scientific Revolutions*, Chicago, IL: University of Chicago Press
Laitin, D. (2003), 'The Perestroikan Challenge to Social Science', *Politics and Society*, 31(1): 163–84
Lieberson, S. (1987), *Making it Count: The Improvement of Social Research and Theory*, Berkeley: University of California Press
Lieberson, S. and F.B. Lynn (2002), 'Barking up the Wrong Branch: Scientific Alternatives to the Current Model of Sociological Science', *Annual Review of Sociology*, 28: 1–19
Lundvall, B.-A., P. Intarakumnerd, and J. Vang, (eds) (2006), *Asia's Innovation Systems in Transition*, Cheltenham: Edward Elgar
Mayer-Schonberger, V. and K. Cukier (2013), *Big Data*, London: John Murray

Maynard Smith, J. (1982), *Evolution and the Theory of Games,* Cambridge: Cambridge University Press
Maynard Smith, J. and E. Szathmary (2000), *The Origins of Life: From the Birth of Life to the Origins of Language,* Oxford: Oxford University Press
McAdam, D., S. Tarrow, and C. Tilly (2001), *Dynamics of Contention,* Cambridge: Cambridge University Press
Palier, B., (ed.) (2010), *A Long Goodbye to Bismarck? The Politics of Welfare Reform in Continental Europe,* Amsterdam: Amsterdam University Press
Palier, B. and C. Martin, (eds) (2008), *Reforming the Bismarckian Welfare Systems,* Oxford: Blackwell
Pierson, P. (2004), *Politics in Time,* Princeton, NJ: Princeton University Press
Popper, K.R. (1994), 'Models, Instruments and Truth: The Status of the Rationality Principle in the Social Sciences', in K.R. Popper (ed.), *The Myth of the Framework: In Defence of Science and Rationality,* London: Routledge: 154–84
Potts, J. (2000), *The New Evolutionary Microeconomics: Complexity, Competence and Adaptive Behaviour,* Cheltenham: Edward Elgar
Powell, J.H. and J.P. Bradford (1998), 'The Security-Strategy Interface: Using Qualitative Process Models to Relate the Security Function to Business Dynamics', *Security Journal,* 10: 151–60
Powell, J.H. and J.P. Bradford (2000), 'Targeting Intelligence Gathering in a Dynamic Competitive Environment', *International Journal of Information Management,* 20: 181–95
Ragin, C.C. (1987), *The Comparative Method,* Berkeley: University of California Press
Ragin, C.C. (2000), *Fuzzy-Set Social Science,* Chicago, IL: University of Chicago Press
Room, G. (2011), *Complexity, Institutions and Public Policy: Agile Decision-Making in a Turbulent World,* Cheltenham: Edward Elgar
Scheffer, M. (2009), *Critical Transitions in Nature and Society,* Princeton, NJ: Princeton University Press
Shubin, N. (2008), *Your Inner Fish,* Harmondsworth: Allen Lane
Skocpol, T. (1979), *States and Social Revolutions,* Cambridge: Cambridge University Press
Sloan Wilson, D. (2008), 'Multilevel Selection Theory and Major Evolutionary Transitions', *Current Directions in Psychological Science,* 17(1): 6–9
Social Exclusion Unit (2004), *The Drivers of Social Exclusion,* London: Office of the Deputy Prime Minister
Solé, R. and J. Bascompte (2006), *Self-Organization in Complex Ecosystems,* Princeton, NJ: Princeton University Press
Stolzenberg, R. (2003), 'Time Matters: On Theory and Method', *Sociological Methods and Research,* 31: 420–7
Streek, W. and K. Thelen, (eds) (2005), *Beyond Continuity: Institutional Change in Advanced Political Economies,* Oxford: Oxford University Press
Tavory, I. and S. Timmermans (2014), *Abductive Analysis: Theorizing Qualitative Research,* Chicago, IL: University of Chicago Press
Thelen, K. (2004), *How Institutions Evolve,* Cambridge: Cambridge University Press
Toner, P. (1999), *Main Currents in Cumulative Causation: The Dynamics of Growth and Development,* London: St Martin's Press
von Bertalanffy, L. (1968), *General System Theory: Foundations, Development, Applications,* New York: George Braziller

Part II
Agile actors

4 Rationality, rationales and agile action

4.1 Introduction

How can we make sense of how social actors probe the complex and turbulent landscapes on which they find themselves? This chapter elaborates the concept of agile action by reference to the established accounts of rational action, by such writers as Weber and Goldthorpe. This provides the basis for examining the rationales of institutions, understood within the larger analysis of political economy. Chapter 5 will then be concerned with the struggles for 'positional advantage' in which agile actors are involved. Chapter 6 offers an analysis of how agile actors – including policy-makers – probe and navigate an uncertain and foggy world.

This all builds on ideas already developed within Part I. The opening chapter was concerned with the relationship between the natural and social sciences – and the contribution to each of the literature on complex systems. In the course of that discussion, it began to engage with the debates around agency and rational action. Chapter 2 was concerned with evolutionary dynamics and their relevance for social science. It emphasised in particular the role of human agency and it introduced the notion of agile action that will be elaborated here. Chapter 3 was likewise concerned with human agency, in historically contingent contexts, and the circumstances under which linear models may be inappropriate.

4.2 Popper on the rationality principle

We start with Popper's exposition of the 'rationality principle' and his application of it to both science and social action. As we shall see, this aligns closely with our own account of agile action and assists in clarifying its relationship to rational action.

Popper (1994: 169) first acknowledges that the 'rationality principle ... has led to countless misunderstandings'; and that 'it has little or nothing to do with the empirical or psychological assertion that man ... in the main ... acts rationally'. He attempts to set matters straight.

He starts with scientific enquiry and progress. He argues that all science begins with problems – and that these problems emerge from dialogue with the tentative solutions to earlier problems. Theories are hunches as to how these new problems might be addressed. He goes on to argue that critical discussion is a device to test such theories for their consistency, both internally and externally, against available knowledge. The rationality of science is simply the rationality of a 'well-conducted critical discussion'.[1]

Here is a clue as to what Popper means when he turns from the rationality of science to that of action. Here he refers to situations where actors are, we might say, also 'well-conducted': that is to say, they are ready to expose themselves to interrogation and critical discussion as to why they did what they did. In other words, actors are ready to *provide a rationale for their actions*, and to have this scrutinised for its internal and external consistency. Indeed, as social actors expose themselves to such scrutiny by others, they tend the more to interrogate and monitor themselves. This is what writers such as Harré and Secord (1972: chs 5–6) take to be the distinguishing and defining feature of what it is to be human: and they consider it central to the generative processes involved in meaningful social action.

Popper also refers to the actor who, far from being well-conducted, acts 'inappropriately' in relation to such questioning. This is an actor who defies the scrutiny we offer, even though we may 'have a wider knowledge of the problem situation' and we can 'interrogate' and demystify it for them. It may be wrong to blame such actors for their incomplete knowledge of their situation; nevertheless, if they are unwilling to question and adjust their rationale, in the face of our efforts to enlighten them, Popper believes this must be a sign of their madness or incompetence. This misses the extent to which the meanings of social situations are contestable (see Section 4.7 below). Writers such as Lukes (2005) might, moreover, point out that even the sane can be locked into mistaken views, for example by the hegemonic cultural power of those around them. Ideological battles are waged precisely as a means of reshaping what counts as a mistaken view, a sign of madness or incompetence.[2]

Popper proceeds to consider what we might mean by 'models' in social science. He argues that these must capture or reconstruct the most typical 'social situations' or 'situational logics'. This is very close to what Weber (1949) says about ideal types. The latter are parsimonious descriptions of some typical social situations in order to bring out their 'situational logic'. Weber's ideal type of the Protestant Ethic provides a good example: embracing as it does the religious mind set of the Puritan and the economic orientation to which – in particular social and historical circumstances – this tended to lead.

We may expect that social actors, when interrogated as to the logic of their actions, will also resort to ideal types such as these. They may, moreover, to some degree impose this logic on what they are doing, in order that their actions are more consistent with the justification they offer. This is the basis on which the sociologist selects appropriate ideal types: for their consistency with the logic of action to which a goodly number of the actors in question are gravitating.

Nevertheless, the sociologist must not lose sight of the fact that these are 'ideal' types: real-world actors will variously diverge from the logical consistency they embody. To this extent, Popper argues, the rationality principle is false as a description of how all or even most people behave (p. 172). Moreover, real-world actors are creative in devising new logics for their courses of action: and this may eventually prompt us as sociologists to adjust our portfolio of ideal types accordingly (Crouch, 2005: chs 2–3).

There is one final element of Popper's discussion that it is worth highlighting: one that again exploits the parallel that he draws between the development of scientific knowledge and the justification of courses of social action. Popper notes that 'we can look upon any particular item of knowledge, and especially upon any scientific theory, as a tentative solution to some problem or other, and as giving rise to new problems' (1994: 156). As scientific or as social actors, we have at our disposal a body of settled knowledge; by taking this as our vantage point we are able to probe problems previously unanticipated; but as we do so, and as we generate further knowledge, it is always possible that the body of settled knowledge with which we started will itself be disturbed. Moreover, at each stage we not only stand on a body of settled knowledge, we also deploy a body of settled procedures and practices, conventions and habits, whether in our scientific community or in the community of our everyday lives. From here we test novel procedures and practices on terrains as yet unexplored; and in due course these may become the new routines of those communities.

We return to this account by Popper of knowledge development and learning, after we have addressed some of the arguments advanced by Goldthorpe.

4.3 Goldthorpe on rational action

Goldthorpe broadly concurs with Popper, as far as the foregoing discussion is concerned. Nevertheless, he also discusses various forms of rational action and their place within sociological explanation. It is on these that we now concentrate. Here, as with Popper, this assists in clarifying our own account of agile action and its relationship to rational and indeed habitual action.

Goldthorpe argues that sociologists should give a privileged status to actions that can be treated 'as being in some sense rational' (2007a: 16). These are actions that to some degree have a coherent logic or rationale: one that can be readily uncovered by appropriate interrogation, as discussed in our treatment of Popper. If such a logic is common to the actions of myriad individuals, albeit with fluctuations around it that are more or less random, the aggregation of these at the macro-level will, Goldthorpe argues, be well captured by that same logic. This will permit the sociologist to explain such macro-level regularities by reference to generative processes that are meaningful at the micro-level.[3]

Goldthorpe (2007a: ch. 16) surveys several variants of rational action theory, in order to identify the forms most suitable for use in sociology, in its quest to explain such regularities. Weber distinguished *zweckrational* (purpose-rational) and *wertrational* (value-rational) action: Goldthorpe has little time for the latter. For Weber's categories of non-rational action – habitual and emotional action – he has even less (Weber, 1947: ch. I). They are little more than background noise.

It is purpose-rational action that Goldthorpe brings centre-stage. 'Actors act rationally when, in the light of well-grounded beliefs, they choose those courses of action that are best calculated to realize their goals' (2007a: 127).[4] Here, the social actor is confronted with a range of options, carrying particular costs, benefits and consequences (2007a: 170). It is, however, unclear whether this purpose-rationality would encompass efforts to reshape the menu of options where this is possible, so as to make them more attractive. For social actors to ignore such possibilities even when they are available – instead, merely adjusting to whatever menu results from the contests of others – would hardly be rational (see Chapter 1 above).[5]

Furthermore, it is unclear whether the actors in Schelling's model (and indeed in that of Hedström) would be counted as purpose-rational (see Chapter 1 above). They follow simple and explicit rules and the rationale for their action is immediately evident. Each of them has a threshold level of tolerance for the proportion of other ethnic groups within their immediate neighbourhood: when that threshold value is exceeded, the resident in question moves elsewhere. This is a simple heuristic, a rule of thumb. It is, therefore, akin to many of the habits and conventions by which we organise and manage our lives – something that both Goldthorpe and Weber would tend to treat as non-rational. Even so, actors can be interrogated for the habits and conventions that they follow; and they can be asked to give a rationale for what they are doing, even if – at the time in question – they were proceeding rather unthinkingly 'on autopilot'.[6] The boundary between rational and habitual is hazier – in principle, not just in practice – than either Goldthorpe or Weber perhaps recognise (but see Goldthorpe, 2007a: 154–5, 178–9).

It is true that in some of the psychological literature, such 'heuristics' are treated as forms of unreflective thinking – and thinking indeed which typically exhibits biases and blunders that are hard-wired into the human psyche (Thaler and Sunstein, 2009; Kahneman, 2011). Such rules of thumb vary considerably, however, and are a matter of learned practice, rather than being just psychological characteristics of the individuals in question. For much of the sociological literature, therefore, such heuristics are better viewed as standard templates carried within the social institutions that surround us: we draw upon them as members of society, adapting them to our particular contexts. They are, moreover, highly consequential: we depend on them for handling the trivia in our lives with an economy of effort, so that we can concentrate our energies on more problematic issues. This rational concentration thus has habit and convention as its necessary counterpart and precondition. Rational action cannot, *pace* Goldthorpe, be privileged in isolation.

Finally, it is also unclear whether Goldthorpe is justified in so readily setting *wertrational* action aside. For Weber *wertrational* action was rational inasmuch as it involved the careful and reflective choice between alternative values and their implications for action: not, it is true, as a means of achieving certain goals, but action that affirmed and lived by the consequences of such a choice. There is no reason why the clarity of such a situational logic need be any less than that which *zweckrational* action embodies.[7]

That is not all. Social actors regularly pose themselves questions of both sorts, albeit to varying degrees, as they make their way in the world, probing the dynamic possibilities that it holds. It is by engaging in such reflection – as to the ends and value commitments they are pursuing, as well as the means they are using to achieve particular goals – that they navigate their world and regularly reassess the rationale for what they are doing.[8] Sociologists who seek to discover the rationale underlying such actions do well to interrogate the actors in question in regards to both.

Having laid out the case for rational action theory, Goldthorpe turns finally to the sorts of data that are likely to be most relevant and illuminating. He seeks to demonstrate an 'elective affinity' between rational action theory (RAT) and the quantitative analysis of large-scale data sets (QAD). It is here, he argues, that sociological theory-building and explanation can best make headway (Goldthorpe, 2007a: ch. 7). Small-scale studies and qualitative case studies are very much a second-best strategy.

He recognises that QAD typically have a rather limited amount of data on each individual respondent. This is the more the case if the QAD, rather than being purpose-built for the enquiry in question, is an 'omnibus' survey designed to serve a wide variety of investigators. Nevertheless, the clearer the question in which the sociologist is interested, the more precisely circumscribed can be the empirical data that are demanded. Goldthorpe argues that a focus on rational action – where this is appropriate – can offer precisely that precision, given the coherence of the logic that it embodies (2007a: 118–27). Nevertheless, small-scale and qualitative case studies may remain a crucial preliminary, in order to establish the rationale or logic of action which the actors in question are typically following.

As we have seen, to establish the rationale of the actions in which individuals are involved may require a process of iterative interrogation. As we saw with Popper, the interrogator may deploy 'his wider knowledge of the problem situation'; and as Goldthorpe similarly argues, this may include the macro-social 'regularities that are not readily apparent to the "lay members" of a society' (2007a: 207). It is for demonstrating such regularities, as an input for interrogations, that QAD is perhaps best-placed. Nevertheless, as we saw in Chapter 1, these regularities may involve non-linear dynamics and be counter-intuitive for the social actors in question. In such cases, social actors may have a clear and coherent logic of individual action, but one whose *Wert-* and *Zweckrationalität* are both then put fundamentally in question, once they are confronted by the relevant macro-social regularities.

4.4 Agile action

Popper focuses upon the *rationale* that underpins a scientific theory or a course of action; the *models* or *ideal types* in which that rationale is captured; and its *critical scrutiny* by the community of other social actors, for its internal and external consistency. As we have seen, he reckons that the 'rationality principle . . . has little or nothing to do with the empirical or psychological assertion that man . . . in the main . . . acts rationally' (p. 169). He, therefore, does not wrestle with the distinction between various sorts of rational and non-rational action. Goldthorpe has no such qualms; he is ready to embrace Popper's arguments for the rationality principle, as set out above; but he also privileges purpose-rational action, as far as sociological explanation is concerned. Here, however, we will argue for 'agile action' as a more appropriate and fundamental conceptual choice (Room, 2011).[9]

Popper draws out the implications of his position for our understanding of the growth of scientific knowledge. The scientific community has at its disposal a body of settled knowledge and practices. By taking this as their vantage point, scientists are able to advance new hunches, probe problems previously unanticipated and test new theories and procedures. These may in due course redefine the knowledge base and routines of the scientific community, reworking or even obliterating the settled knowledge of old.

As we have seen, what Popper says of scientists he then applies also to social actors. No less than scientists, communities of social actors have a settled body of knowledge and habits, albeit frequently contested and reworked, and varying between different social milieux. With these as their starting point, social actors are able to probe problems previously unanticipated, terrains as yet unexplored; and from this new position, to articulate new alternatives to that settled body. For this they must deploy mental models as to how the world will unfold; the more so, when they are faced with fellow actors who are also trying to probe and reshape that world. How actors probe – and with what results – will of course depend on the resources at their disposal, the vantage point which they enjoy and the power that they can exercise.

In all this, the role of the social scientist is to enhance the critical scrutiny and interrogation to which social actors subject themselves and each other: testing the consistency and coherence of the rationales they provide for their actions and obliging them to make those rationales explicit. This will, on the one hand, be concerned with the settled body of habits and conventions in which social actors are immersed and which they take for granted, until interrogation leads to their conscious articulation; and, on the other hand, with agile actions that probe and explore new problems and dilemmas, where actors are in general more reflective and deliberate. This interrogation by the social scientist typically includes watching and listening, as social actors interrogate each other and contest each other's accounts (Tavory and Timmermans, 2014: ch. 4).[10]

Nevertheless, if social actors are to probe new problems, this is possible only from the security of that settled body of habits and conventions. Between habitual and agile action there is therefore a dual connection. First, the cognitive economy in the former leaves maximum energy for the latter. Second, however, we must recognise that, empirically, which matters are handled in which way is itself fluid. It is when actors detect anomalous patterns, including for example those that fall outside certain critical thresholds, that this alerts them to the need for an agile rather than a habitual response. These are commonly situations that present opportunities or threats for the actors in question, and that may indeed be of major existential significance. This relationship between habitual and agile action is therefore fluid and it will vary between actors, depending on their interests and the resources and positional leverage of which they dispose (for a somewhat parallel discussion, see Nelson and Winter (1982: ch. 5)).

Our conceptual preference for 'agile' over 'rational' action springs also from the account of social dynamics which was offered in Chapter 1. There we argued that it was insufficient to treat the macro-regularities that we observe in empirical data sets as the linear aggregation of myriad micro-choices. Social actors not only act, they also interact, and this can set non-linear processes in motion, producing the macro-patterns that we observe. It is from these non-linearities that the anomalous patterns to which we have just referred – the threats and opportunities – not infrequently emerge. Indeed, social actors commonly search for these transformative macro-dynamics, probing how to reshape their direction. It may have been the complexity literature that inspired that account in Chapter 1, but it is also, as we have now seen, consistent with Popper's account of the growth of knowledge.

Agile action is thus a theory of action which – much more than 'purpose-rational action' – captures the dynamic interrelationship of micro to macro that we presented in Chapter 1: and upon which the rest of this book will build. It also accommodates our suggestion that as they make their way in the world, probing the dynamic possibilities that it holds, social actors will regularly pose themselves and each other questions as to both the *Wert-* and *Zweckrationalität* of their actions, as a means of navigating and leveraging that world: and that the sociologist will need to interrogate them in regards to both. This is not 'purpose-rational' in the sense of 'instrumental': but it *is* indeed action which is both *purposive* and has a *rationale*.[11]

4.5 Varieties of action theory

It is from this standpoint that we can compare and contrast the principal forms of rational action theory that are in use: or, better, the principal theories of *purposive action with a rationale*. As Goldthorpe (2007a: ch. 7) notes, these differ significantly, notwithstanding some family resemblances. We distinguish three main approaches.

First, social actors may be seen as *calculators of utility*. They are confronted with a range of options, carrying particular costs, benefits and consequences, by reference to which such calculations are made (Goldthorpe, 2007a: 170). This is central to rational choice theory. Beyond such calculation, there is hardly any reference to purposive action: including action aimed, for example, at reshaping the menu of options which are available and their respective costs and benefits. Nor is there much attention to the institutional framework and setting within which such costs and benefits sit.[12]

Second, social actors may be seen as *followers of rules*: albeit the rationale for following particular rules may be somewhat hidden even to the actors in question, becoming evident only in response to interrogation and the reflection that this provokes. Here there is little reference to action aimed at reshaping the rules and their fields of application. This has been central to our discussion of habitual action: highlighting the settled body of knowledge and practices that such habits embody, the rules of thumb by which we manage much of our daily lives. Nevertheless, they may also be oppressive and coercive and driven by the interests of others. Sociologists who interrogate the rationale for such rules may, therefore, raise questions about their legitimacy and about the institutional and political context within which they are sustained and enforced (Lukes, 2005).

Third, social actors may be seen as *agile probers and re-weavers of their world*. They pursue purposes beyond mere conformity with the existing rules. They test and break, circumvent and rework these rules, in order to have a chance of achieving those larger purposes (Crouch, 2005). They may invent new rules, borrow and apply those from other fields, or recycle the *bricolage* of the past. They probe the purposes and plans of other actors, whether to cooperate or to defeat them. In all this they seek to mobilise transformative dynamic synergies of the sort we discussed in Chapters 1 and 3 above. Sociologists who seek the rationale for such actions will need to interrogate the actors in question about both the *Wert-* and the *Zweckrationalität* of what they are doing. Indeed, social actors regularly pose for themselves and each other questions of both sorts, albeit in varying degrees, as they make their way in the world, probing the dynamic possibilities that it holds. Nevertheless, the existing rules and habits provide the essential solid ground, without which there would be no base – however provisional and contestable – from which to probe the new: albeit from that new vantage point they may then rearrange the settled ground from which they came.

Depending on the settled body of knowledge and practices on which they draw, social actors are liable to respond in radically different ways to similar opportunities or threats. This, for example, is central to Weber's sociology of religion, and his account of the quite different orientations to both political and economic activity which occidental and oriental religions tend to produce (Weber, 1965). What this underlines is the importance of taking into account the communities and collectivities where people develop and perpetuate these shared meanings (see, for example, Heath *et al.*, 2013: ch. 6).

Gladwell (2008) offers vivid case studies of how such legacies shape the range of responses which people make to novel situations. Safety requires that aircrews on civilian flights employ a high level of teamwork and mutual correction when errors are made. In the case of Korea, however, traditions of deference prevailed even in the cockpit, with catastrophic levels of air crashes during the period when the national airline was establishing itself. Only by extracting the personnel in question from that Korean context and retraining them, in an Anglophone medium and culture, were the effects of this legacy overcome. In the same book, Gladwell also describes the 'culture of honour' that prevailed among small rural communities in the highlands of Kentucky during the nineteenth century and the pattern of belligerent responses to insults. Such responses continue to prevail among the modern descendants of those highlanders, as they interact in professional contexts within urban America, with sometimes explosive consequences.

The understandings and practices with which people operate may thus produce consequences that under interrogation they would disavow. Popper anticipates that except for the insane, interrogation will lead to the necessary corrections, whether this refers to our scientific or our social lives. This may be overly simplistic. Lukes (2005) warns that the everyday meanings and habits with which we operate are constructed in part by powerful actors, in disregard of our own interests. It is only by making sense of the world in which social actors find themselves, which they interrogate and navigate, modify and manage, that we can understand the courses of action in which they are engaged and the rationale that it has for them. This goes to the heart of what Weber (1947: ch. 1) discussed in terms of *verstehende Soziologie*.

Here, then, are three sharply contrasting conceptualisations of social action. Nevertheless, as we have seen, agile action presupposes that much of our action is habitual, supported by a settled body of knowledge and practices. The social actor as rule breaker and maker presupposes the social actor as rule taker and follower. What then of the social actor as a calculator of utility? It is true that agile action involves careful reflection as to the *Wert-* and *Zweckrationalität* of these actions: this in turn will involve consideration of trade-offs and the consequences of different directions of action: the calculation of utility might well constitute one form and moment in that assessment. Nevertheless, to reduce our analysis of social action to this is hardly justified by the analytical pay-off it affords.

4.6 Agile action and the rationale of institutions

We have argued that if social actors are to probe new problems and possibilities, this is possible only from the security of a settled body of habits and conventions, involving rules of thumb and standard templates. These are best understood, not as psychological characteristics of the individuals in question, but as a matter of learned practice, carried within the social institutions that surround us. In probing the rationale for action, therefore, we also and unavoidably interrogate the rationale for the institutions in which social actors find themselves enmeshed and whose possibilities of transformation they explore. This has of course long been a central element of the sociological tradition.

We turn now to consider the place of institutions in the foregoing account of agile action. Once again, it is useful to recall the 'two sociologies' distinguished by Dawe (1970): the 'sociology of order' and the 'sociology of control'. For the former, the macro-level is a fixed, exogenous and more or less coherent 'context', constraining the micro-behaviour of individual actors. The 'sociology of order' is concerned, therefore, with the normative and institutional structures that dominate our lives, enforcing the rules of our interactions and giving or denying authority to the choices we make. This is consistent with writers such as North (1990: ch. 1), understanding institutions in terms of the rules of social interaction they embody. These rules shape the patterns of action and group formation that can develop, and the organisation of competence and knowledge that can be deployed.

A large sociological and political science literature, couched in these terms, is concerned with the diversity of institutions and the different sets of rules that they embody. Scharpf (1997), for example, distinguishes several ideal types: the 'institutional minimalism' of the market; hierarchical coordination 'in the shadow of the State'; and various forms of network and association governed by negotiated agreements.[13] Ostrom (1990) examines cooperative institutions, as an alternative both to markets and to hierarchical direction by the State, and often more effective for the management of 'common pool resources'. A similar three-fold distinction is evident in Etzioni's analysis of modes of organisational compliance: instrumental, coercive and moral (Etzioni, 1961).

We also recall the sociological literature concerned with the meso-level of communities and collectivities, where social contacts may shape the values, identities, meanings and hopes that individuals embrace: and indeed their prejudices, which *pace* Schelling may not be given and fixed (Heath *et al.*, 2013: ch. 6). This means not just residential communities but also, for example, workplace and occupational communities (Fox, 1971).

The 'sociology of control' is, in contrast, concerned with the efforts of social actors to construct and reconstruct the institutional fabric within which they find themselves and to impose their meanings and purposes upon it. Modern societies offer a multiplicity of institutional terrains, with most actors involved in many of them simultaneously. There are commonly trade-offs between the goals pursued on one terrain and those pursued on another; and there may be scope for cooperation or conflict, not just within individual terrains but across them. Just as important, the outcome of interactions on one terrain may affect the resources which each actor can then bring to the struggle on another; or indeed, whether they can even gain access. On some terrains, a variety of institutional settings may be in play and can be variously invoked by the social actors concerned (Crouch, 2005). This may also permit venue or forum 'shopping', as actors choose where and how to pursue a given set of goals.[14] Here again, actors differ, both in their power to make use of such opportunities and in the skill and creativity with which they do so.

The 'sociology of order' directs our attention to the habits and rules of thumb that are carried within the social institutions that surround us and which we follow rather unthinkingly in our everyday lives. The 'sociology of control', in contrast, directs attention to the efforts of agile social actors to probe and construct *new* institutional possibilities (or to contest and resist the attempts by others to do so). Here institutions are construed not as the normative structures which enforce the rules of our interactions, but as the connective tissue which agile social actors re-weave, as they probe and shape the transformative dynamics of their world.

Institutions provide *the robust connections required for this imperative coordination* (Weber, 1947: Part III). They enable social actors to mobilise people, technologies, finance and other resources, combining and redeploying them in new directions, in a timely and predictable manner. Goldthorpe, for example, in his analysis of social class, brings centre-stage the forms of imperative coordination to which different groups of workers are subject: whether this is a labour contract, involving extrinsic monetary rewards, or a service contract, through which the individual is offered a 'career' of steady occupational advance (Bukodi et al., 2015). Brynjolffson and Coleman examine the dramatically expanded potential for coordination that is offered by the new information technologies: whether this involves businesses rapidly scaling up their operations, in the 'weightless' economy (Brynjolfsson et al., 2006), or hackers commandeering networks of computers as instruments for their attacks (Coleman, 2014: ch. 4).

Institutions carry *competing meanings and 'definitions of the situation'*. It is by reference to these diverse affiliations that individuals craft their identities and seek to provide a connected rationale for their lives.[15] It is also around these competing meanings that we collectively mobilise and that struggles for institutional change are therefore waged. This struggle is concerned with the alternative values by reference to which we live our lives: what we earlier discussed in terms of the *Wertrationalität* of our actions.

Institutions also carry competing *memories* – and the emotional attachments to particular communities and identities that these involve. See, for example, Deák's discussion of the painful memories and moral ambivalence with which the occupied countries of Europe had to grapple post-1945 and the tangled social divisions which the occupation bequeathed (Deák et al., 2000). Institutions also carry competing *hopes* (Coleman, 2014: 395–400). These meanings, memories and hopes are then the basis of competing *moral claims*, as social actors contest or defend their social world (Frye, 2012). They can all be interrogated for their rationale: and all may then figure in our explanations of social action.

Social actors draw on networks of *distributed intelligence* to obtain *early information about threats and opportunities* – with weak ties more useful than strong ties for tapping into distant signals (Granovetter, 1973). From here they also draw mental models as to how the world is likely to unfold. These networks also are part of the institutional connections of society (Christakis and Fowler, 2009). This is a logic of cooperation and communication. Such cooperation is as central to the notion of agile action as abstract individualism is to rational choice (much of the literature on which ignores the community context of social actors: see Heath et al. (2013)).

This cooperation may involve actors who differ greatly in their *interests* and in *the power and advantage* of which they dispose. (Much of the literature concerned with cooperation among rational self-interested actors likewise makes little or no reference to differences in power.) Big actors can provide smaller actors with connections and intelligence – a shortcut to a larger universe. They can provide islands of stability: the settled body of habits and conventions that smaller actors need if they are to probe the novelties of their world. This can also mean incorporation of those smaller actors into their domains on adverse terms: a stable but oppressive order with little scope for such creativity. Big actors may also disrupt and destabilise the world of those smaller actors, offloading the costs of uncertainty onto them. Here all that may be left is to 'hunker down' and await whatever may happen. This is why any analysis of social action and institutions must be set within an understanding of political economy and the larger socio-political settlement.

88 *Agile actors*

Even so, no big actor is ever wholly secure; there is always scope for others to undermine and rework the institutional tissue and the forms of imperative coordination it embodies (Scott, 1998: 351). Indeed, the more extensive the terrain that a big actor dominates, and the more scaled-up the modes of coordination that it applies, the more attractive the target that it offers, and the more costly the consequences if that domain is successfully invaded. Small intruders may align with big actors, the better to invade that domain and develop transformative dynamic synergies of their own. Thus guerrilla armies frame their tactics by reference to those of the army they confront (Harford, 2011: 244); and small companies may welcome incorporation by multinationals, as enabling them, to some degree, to take over from below (Kristensen and Zeitlin, 2005). It is, we might say, from their own imperial garments that the funeral shroud of these big actors is woven by those who go on to displace them.[16]

4.7 Conclusion

We live in a social world of partially decomposed systems – in other words, a world each of whose components interact with only a limited number of others (Simon, 1969: ch. 8). This, we have seen, makes for a lot of stability and predictability, but also some uncertainty and turbulence. The argument of the present chapter resonates with that of its predecessors.

Chapter 1 was centrally concerned with micro-level interactions among social actors: with the non-linear macro-dynamics that can then emerge: and with the counter-intuitive macro-level patterns that result. It looked in part to the complexity literature for an understanding of these. Chapter 3 was concerned with the General Linear Model and the difficulties posed by interactions among the variables. These can, to some degree, be dealt with through smart technical 'fixes': nevertheless, deeper ontological and conceptual questions are raised. It was in those circumstances that we argued for the 'contingent historical model' instead.

The present chapter has been concerned with 'agile action' – seen in relation to habitual action and the various forms of rational action that we find in the social scientific literature. Habitual action involves conventions and rules of thumb that are discrete to particular areas of our everyday lives: areas which must be stable and settled if such rules are to 'work' in a predictable fashion. These areas must, therefore, have only very limited interactions – no less than the social actors of Chapter 1, or the variables of the GLM. It is when that condition no longer applies – and when there is, therefore, turbulence and uncertainty – that social actors can no longer rely on habits and conventions, and must instead be 'agile', probing and testing the dynamic possibilities that this unsettled ground holds.

As in previous chapters, we have here underlined the central place of purposeful struggle and contested meaning-making. Interactions between social actors and processes – and between the variables by which our social science models seek to capture these – are shaped by the powerful. This is why we have situated the discussion of agile action within an analysis of institutional dynamics and political economy. To interrogate that political economy and to understand its rationale is therefore central to the task of social science.

The present chapter began with Popper's 'rationality principle'. This involves interrogating actors and calling them to account, for the consistency and coherence of the rationale they provide for their actions. There is, however, another sense in which they may also be called to account: and indeed, it is arguable that the two senses are inextricably linked. This second sense is accountability for their exercise of power. This is a key part of the argument that Lukes makes, in his re-analysis of the concept of power in political sociology: and it is an argument to which Hayward in particular has returned in the ongoing debate with Lukes (Lukes, 2005; Hayward, 2006).

Lukes and Hayward distinguish two ways in which we can hold power-holders to account. There is, on the one hand, the 'backward-looking' attribution of blame or credit for the present situation. There is also, however, the 'forward-looking' attribution of responsibility for addressing that situation henceforth: on the part of 'politically responsible agents, in strategic positions, who are able to make a difference' (Lukes, 2006: 172). This is the realm of public policy.

It is with this that the third section of this book will be concerned. In particular, it will examine public policy in terms of the settled ground which it provides for citizens and the ways in which it enables them to probe creatively the world around them. It will, in other words, build on our discussion of agile action in this chapter, as well as on our discussion of complex social dynamics in Part I. It is after all not uncommon for social scientists to allow their understanding of social actors to frame the questions they pose in regards to society and public policy: we will make this somewhat more explicit than is often the case. From that vantage point we will also reflect critically on these competing understandings of social action and the assumptions about public policy which they carry with them.

Notes

1 There are parallels between Popper's argument here and those of Kuhn (1970) and Collingwood (1942).
2 In the 1970s, it used to be said that members of the UK Conservative Party were deeply divided in their views of Sir Keith Joseph, who was Margaret Thatcher's mentor in thinking about shrinking the State. Half of them reckoned he was mad, whereas the rest thought he was 'stark staring bonkers'. However, that 'madness' eventually became the conventional wisdom, and not just within the Conservative Party.
3 Goldthorpe has a separate essay on the relationship between sociological and historical enquiry, in which he contrasts the sort of evidence deployed in the two cases (2007a: ch. 2). Sociology commonly involves the collection of fieldwork evidence provided by the living, which can in principle be supplemented by repeat visits, as the sociologist's enquiries unfold, and the theoretical questions that are posed perhaps shift. In the case of history, however, the evidence inheres in the 'relics' left by those now dead: here no repeat visits are possible. For living respondents, therefore, interrogation may serve to modify their actions, as they reflect on them. Historical subjects are immune to such revision. However, that is not the end of the matter. The reason

why historical subjects are of interest is in providing insights into the purposes and struggles that wove the social fabric within which today's living actors find themselves enmeshed (Collingwood, 1942). This, of course, is key to the contingent historical model (CHM) which we set out in Chapter 3, as an alternative to the General Linear Model (GLM).

4 This choice by Goldthorpe is also appropriate, given some of the specific scholarly battles in which he has been engaged: in particular to challenge explanations of working-class low achievement by reference to their cultural values. Here he has been at pains to demonstrate that working-class aspirations – and their awareness of what different occupations offer – are little different from those of middle-class homes: but that they are also well aware that their chances of attaining those more desirable occupations are small, given the social and economic barriers that they face (Goldthorpe, 2007b: ch. 7).

5 It is also unclear how far this version of purpose-rationality can encompass rationales set within a game-theoretic (rather than a decision-theoretic) framework. The latter involves behaviour that is contingent on expectations of what other actors will do: strategic opponents who may be skilled in concealing their intentions (Jervis, 1997: 85).

6 Under interrogation, actors can provide a rationale even for habitual actions, as they reflect upon them and bring them to consciousness. This could perhaps take either of two forms: 'I went through the green light because this is what the highway code stipulates'; or 'I went through the green light because of the habits I developed when I first learned to drive'. Either way, the action in question did not at the time involve the actor thinking carefully about means or ends or consequences; but it *was* possible for the actor to be challenged and interrogated subsequently, and asked to provide a rationale for what he or she did rather unthinkingly at the time. Moreover, the interrogation might involve the sociologist challenging the internal or external consistency of the justificatory narrative – for example, by pointing out that the policeman who this morning stood at the road junction was clearly expecting drivers to heed him, rather than obeying the lights; or that the driver who is being interrogated, far from being on 'autopilot', had let out a 'Whoopy!' of delight, as the policeman leapt aside to escape being killed.

7 For example, as already noted, there was for Weber a very clear logic and coherence between the Puritan's religious beliefs, the existential insecurities that flowed from these and the energy with which the Puritan then threw himself into his business enterprise. This was captured in the statistical association that Weber established between Protestantism and the bearers of the capitalist work ethic. This did not require Weber to make any judgement as to how reasonable or well-grounded were the beliefs themselves.

8 'Goal' is a somewhat ambiguous term. It may refer to levels of income and consumption – my goal is to earn £50k a year – or to a trajectory of self-development and fulfilment. The first will tend to pose questions about the *Zweckrationalität* of actions – was it really sensible to take a job as a postman, if £50k was the goal? The latter in contrast will tend to pose questions about the *Wertrationalität* of action – was it sensible to combine the ambition to raise a family with the decision to enter a highly competitive and entrepreneurial work environment?

9 The notion of agile action is far from novel. For examples of very similar positions, see Schön (1987: ch. 2) on 'reflection-in-action', Scott (1998: ch. 9) on 'metis' and Crouch (2005) on 'institutional entrepreneurs'.

10 Tavory and Timmermans (2014) offer an approach to social science similar to that of Popper, drawing upon Peirce and the pragmatists in particular. They consider first (Chapter 4) how social scientists become adept in putting the habitual and familiar social world in question, so as to illuminate its counter-intuitive patterns and anomalies: 'surprises' in relation to which they can then develop new hunches. To develop such perceptual insight – the ability to view the familiar from new standpoints – typically

presupposes a wide theoretical repertoire and the skill to re-weave and apply this to new problems. It can also be developed by study of – and involvement in – a wide variety of social actions.

On this basis, Tavory and Timmermans argue, social scientists will be able to interrogate social actors, testing the consistency and coherence of the rationales they offer for their actions – and pressing them to make those rationales explicit. They will also, however, watch and listen to the ways that social actors engage with each other, interrogating and contesting each other's accounts and negotiating the meanings that they variously give to their world. This includes noticing how actors 'talk past' each other, missing each other's meanings but also purposely contesting and side-lining them. Causal explanation will then treat this 'spiral' of meaning-making not as random noise around some version of rational action, as proposed by Goldthorpe, but rather as contested efforts to weave social processes and connections together.

11 If this conceptualisation of 'agile action' is of any value, it can be expected to resonate with elements of the extensive debates on social action that we find in the social science literature. I deal with a number of these, but I cannot deal with them all and I must leave that to other scholars, if they find it fruitful. Thus, for example, I am aware that there may be meat here for Bourdieu scholars to get their teeth into, particularly in relation to his notion of 'habitus'. Scholars of critical realism may likewise consider how useful 'agile action' is, for example in relation to Archer's account of reflexivity and routines (Archer, 2010). Notice, however, that I understand reflexivity in relation to the critical scrutiny and interrogation to which social actors subject themselves and each other, testing the rationales they provide for their actions. Notice also my stress on the transformative macro-dynamics for which social actors commonly search and whose direction they seek to reshape: what Chapter 1 described as *transformative* realism. Finally, these are all to be understood by reference to the distribution of power, set within a larger institutional analysis of political economy.

12 This focus on the calculation of utility is in part the legacy of Richard von Neumann, who made groundbreaking contributions to both linear programming and rational choice theory.

13 It is, of course, a matter of debate, as to how 'minimal' are the institutional underpinnings that markets require, with mainstream economists heavily criticised by institutional economists, political scientists and sociologists, for under-estimating this (Polanyi, 1944).

14 As Jones and Sergot (1996) point out, this is most obvious in quasi-legal situations, where a given case may potentially fall under a variety of different legal provisions, and where the choice of the appropriate legal basis can have fateful consequences. Such forum shopping has been given considerable attention in the international relations literature, where overlapping but fragmented mandates among the various international organisations of the modern era offer plenty of scope for such creativity (Davis, 2006). This work on venue shopping is part of a larger international relations literature concerned with two-level games (Evans *et al.*, 1993).

15 Goldthorpe and Lockwood's studies of the Affluent Worker centre on his search for precisely this sort of coherent meaning for his working career (Goldthorpe *et al.*, 1969). See also the discussion by Tavory and Timmermans (2014: ch. 5) of 'intersituational variation' as illustrated by urban ethnographies such as those by Whyte and Liebow.

16 This, Coleman argues, is why large corporations welcome Anonymous hackers, as a test of the resilience of their systems. They even solicit contributions from Anonymous to their own future-scanning, their efforts to anticipate possible disruptive change. This is how Anonymous, even in its attacks on corporations, in some degree becomes part of their network of distributed intelligence, alerting them to how the world is likely to unfold (Coleman, 2014: ch. 8).

References

Archer, M.S. (2010), 'Routine, Reflexivity and Realism', *Sociological Theory*, 28(3): 272–303

Brynjolfsson, E.J., A. McFee, F. Zhu, and M. Sorell (2006), *Scale Without Mass: Business Process Replication and Industry Dynamics*, Harvard Business School Technology and Operations Management Unit Research Paper No 07–016

Bukodi, E., J.H. Goldthorpe, L. Waller, and J. Kuha (2015), 'The Mobility Problem in Britain: New Findings from the Analysis of Birth Cohort Data', *The British Journal of Sociology*, 66(1): 93–117

Christakis, N. and J. Fowler (2009), *Connected: The Amazing Power of Social Networks and How They Change our Lives*, London: HarperPress

Coleman, G. (2014), *Hacker, Hoaxer, Whistleblower, Spy: The Many Faces of Anonymous*, London: Verso

Collingwood, R.G. (1942), *The Idea of History*, Oxford: Oxford University Press

Crouch, C. (2005), *Capitalist Diversity and Change: Recombinant Governance and Institutional Entrepreneurs*, Oxford: Oxford University Press

Davis, C. (2006), *The Politics of Forum Choice for Trade Disputes*, Philadelphia: American Political Science Association, 31 August

Dawe, A. (1970), 'The Two Sociologies', *British Journal of Sociology*, 21(2): 207–18

Deák, I., J.T. Gross, and T. Judt, (eds) (2000), *The Politics of Retribution in Europe*, Princeton, NJ: Princeton University Press

Etzioni, A. (1961), *Complex Organisations*, New York: Free Press

Evans, P.B., H.K. Jackson, and R.D. Putnam (1993), *Double-Edged Diplomacy: International Bargaining and Domestic Politics*, Berkeley: University of California Press

Fox, A. (1971), *A Sociology of Work in Industry*, London: Collier-Macmillan

Frye, M. (2012), 'Bright Futures in Malawi's New Dawn: Educational Aspirations as Assertions of Identity', *American Journal of Sociology*, 117(6): 1565–624

Gladwell, M. (2008), *Outliers: The Story of Success*, London: Penguin

Goldthorpe, J.H. (2007a), *On Sociology (2nd edition): Volume One: Critique and Program*, Stanford, CA: Stanford University Press

Goldthorpe, J.H. (2007b), *On Sociology (2nd edition): Volume Two: Illustrations and Retrospect*, Stanford, CA: Stanford University Press

Goldthorpe, J.H., D. Lockwood, F. Bechhofer, and J. Platt (1969), *The Affluent Worker in the Class Structure*, Cambridge: Cambridge University Press

Granovetter, M. (1973), 'The Strength of Weak Ties', *American Journal of Sociology*, 78: 1360–80

Harford, T. (2011), *Adapt: Why Success Always Starts with Failure*, London: Little, Brown

Harré, R. and P.F. Secord (1972), *The Explanation of Social Behaviour*, Oxford: Blackwell

Hayward, C.R. (2006), 'On Power and Responsibility', *Political Studies Review*, 4(2): 156–63

Heath, A., S.D. Fisher, G. Rosenblatt, D. Sanders, and M. Sobolewska (2013), *The Political Integration of Ethnic Minorities in Britain*, Oxford: Oxford University Press

Jervis, R. (1997), *System Effects: Complexity in Political and Social Life*, Princeton, NJ: Princeton University Press

Jones, A. and M. Sergot (1996), 'A Formal Characterisation of Institutionalised Power', *Journal of the IGPL*, 4: 429–45

Kahneman, D. (2011), *Thinking, Fast and Slow*, London: Allen Lane

Kristensen, P.H. and J. Zeitlin (2005), *Local Players in Global Games: The Strategic Constitution of a Multinational Corporation,* Oxford: Oxford University Press

Kuhn, T.S. (1970), *The Structure of Scientific Revolutions,* Chicago, IL: University of Chicago Press

Lukes, S.M. (2005), *Power: A Radical View (Second Edition),* Basingstoke: Palgrave Macmillan

Lukes, S.M. (2006), 'Reply to Comments', *Political Studies Review,* 4(2): 164–73

Nelson, R. and S. Winter (1982), *An Evolutionary Theory of Economic Change,* Cambridge, MA: Harvard University Press

North, D.C. (1990), *Institutions, Institutional Change and Economic Performance,* Cambridge: Cambridge University Press

Ostrom, E. (1990), *Governing the Commons: The Evolution of Institutions for Collective Action,* Cambridge: Cambridge University Press

Polanyi, K. (1944), *The Great Transformation,* New York: Rinehart

Popper, K.R. (1994), 'Models, Instruments and Truth: The Status of the Rationality Principle in the Social Sciences', in K.R. Popper (ed.), *The Myth of the Framework: In Defence of Science and Rationality,* London: Routledge: 154–84

Room, G. (2011), *Complexity, Institutions and Public Policy: Agile Decision-Making in a Turbulent World,* Cheltenham: Edward Elgar

Scharpf, F.W. (1997), *Games Real Actors Play: Actor-Centred Institutionalism in Policy Research,* Boulder, CO: Westview Press

Schön, D.A. (1987), *Educating the Reflective Practitioner,* San Francisco, CA: Jossey-Bass Publishers

Scott, J.C. (1998), *Seeing Like a State,* Newhaven, CT: Yale University Press

Simon, H.A. (1969), *The Sciences of the Artificial,* Cambridge, MA: MIT Press

Tavory, I. and S. Timmermans (2014), *Abductive Analysis: Theorizing Qualitative Research,* Chicago, IL: University of Chicago Press

Thaler, R.H. and C.R. Sunstein (2009), *Nudge: Improving Decisions about Health Wealth, and Happiness (Revised edition),* London: Penguin

Weber, M. (1947), *The Theory of Social and Economic Organization,* New York: Free Press

Weber, M. (1949), *The Methodology of the Social Sciences,* New York: Free Press

Weber, M. (1965), *The Sociology of Religion,* London: Methuen (first published in German, 1922)

5 Positional advantage
A three-dimensional analysis

5.1 Introduction

From the opening chapters of this book, we have made frequent reference to positional advantage and the positional struggles in which social actors are involved. Chapter 1 argued that in applying complexity perspectives to the social world, it was essential to acknowledge such struggles and the exercise of power that they involve. Positional advantage was central to Chapter 2, elaborating the 'dance' between artificial and natural selection; to Chapter 3, arguing for 'contingent historical development'; and to Chapter 4, concerned with agile action. It is time to give more attention to this notion.

This chapter argues that the concept of *positional advantage* can provide significant analytical leverage in social science, but that it has been rather neglected since the work of Hirsch (1977). The chapter aims to make good that deficit by clarifying the concept and demonstrating its relevance for a range of social scientific debates. It takes stock of the various intellectual traditions within which positional advantage finds a place; and it offers a conceptual vantage point from which they may be viewed more systematically than has been achieved hitherto.

When we speak of 'advantage' as the goal of social actors, we mean advantage *relative to others*. This is not of course the only goal of social actors. They also seek mastery of their physical environment; and they seek to fill their bellies and find shelter from the elements. But even in pursuing these goals, the pursuit of advantage over others is seldom wholly absent.

By *positional* advantage we mean advantage that actors have by virtue of the positions that they occupy (as distinct, for example, by virtue of the possession of personal talents or money). To say a 'position' implies that there is some *structure*; that there are *positions* in this structure; that from such positions benefits are available that would not otherwise be so; and that to occupy this position gives the occupier some security of tenure, in face of rivals. By occupying a particular position, I enjoy access to status, political power and material benefits and I can exclude you from them, or at least shape the terms on which you access them. There is no implication that such structures and positions are fixed and unchanging.

This is consistent with the broad mainstream of sociological literature during recent decades. Take, for example, the review by Goldthorpe and Bevan (1977) of the literature on social stratification in Britain. They take stratification as involving unequal advantage and power, as manifested in structures of hierarchical differentiation and underpinned by institutional arrangements. As they note, advantage and power are closely interrelated: advantage being possession of, or control over, whatever is generally valued, and power being the capacity to bring about that possession or control. 'Advantage' is thus a distributional aspect of stratification, while 'power' is relational. Therefore, while the focus of this chapter is on positional advantage – access to and control over positions that grant whatever is generally valued – it will inevitably also have implications for debates on power (including, for example, Lukes (2005)).

Nevertheless, the foregoing could leave us with a somewhat limited and static notion of 'position' and 'advantage'. Contrast this with the notion of 'mechanical advantage' as used by physicists, referring for example to levers or pulleys, and to the way in which these amplify the force that can be applied. Or contrast it with the notion of 'adversarial advantage' that is used in cryptography, to measure the scope for an intruder to by-pass or neutralise security controls. It is with the leverage that positions afford their occupants, and the scope that this brings them for contesting and transforming social arrangements, that we shall be primarily concerned. In terms of Dawe's classic distinction, this is inspired more by a sociology of action and control, rather than a sociology of order (Dawe, 1970).

To speak of a struggle for positional advantage does not preclude cooperation: on the contrary, social actors are hardly able to secure positional advantage over some without first securing cooperation from others. The previous chapter considered at some length the forms of coordination that are mediated through institutions, and the various forms of compliance that these may involve. There is also scope for altruistic solidarity and mutual aid. Indeed, as we will see in the conclusion to this chapter, it is to such sentiments that Hirsch implicitly appeals, in part at least, when arguing for public policies that will reduce positional struggle to a level that will avoid excessive social conflict.

This chapter starts by offering a conceptual vantage point from which positional advantage may be viewed, in terms of three dimensions. It demonstrates the analytical relevance of this for a range of social scientific debates, notably those concerned with the concept of power and with the application of evolutionary perspectives in social dynamics. It concludes by revisiting the policy inferences drawn in Hirsch's original essay.

5.2 The one-dimensional view: positional advantage as a pecking order

Hirsch (1977) provides an influential account of positional advantage in relation to the distribution of life chances. One of his illustrations is of a crowd at a football match or other spectator event. If a few people stand on tiptoe they will get a better view over the other spectators' heads. If, however, everyone else also then stands on tiptoe, that early advantage is quickly nullified.

Hirsch applies this idea to what he terms the 'positional economy' and 'positional goods'.[1] These are goods that confer benefit only insofar as they improve a person or group's position relative to that of others. To some degree at least, educational credentials may have this character, if they are sought not for the intrinsic value of the learning they embody, but as part of a competition for entry to elite occupations.[2] Unlike the 'material economy', the distribution of fruits in the 'positional economy' is therefore a zero-sum game. Hirsch sought clear distributional principles – not just in theoretical terms but as a matter of practical politics – for such positional goods, so as to avoid an ever-intensifying but ultimately self-defeating competition.

For Hirsch, therefore, positional advantage involves the establishing, contesting and maintaining of a pecking order. This we refer to as the *one-dimensional view of positional advantage*.

Hirsch makes no assumption that this positional competition is run on equal terms. The terms on which today's competition unfolds may well be shaped by the outcome of yesterday's competition. Indeed, instead of fighting with yesterday's winners, it may be best to leave them to occupy the dominant positions and then fight for what is left.[3]

Hirsch also recognises that positional advantage today may soon dissipate. To stand on tiptoe brings advantage: those behind you can offset the disadvantage you impose on them, by also standing on tiptoe, without diminishing your advantage; but you and they are vulnerable to anyone further to the front who chooses to stand on tiptoe. But once the game has finished, it is those at the front who may be at a disadvantage, in the race for the pub or the bus.

Similarly, your educational credentials may have won you a job, but others with stronger credentials who arrive later may be able to dislodge you. You may be able to appeal to legal rules or social conventions (such as rules of 'first in, last out' at work), to discourage others from mounting such a challenge; but the struggle to maintain your prized position will demand eternal vigilance. Meanwhile, however, that prize may fall in value, as jobs once core to an enterprise become marginalised, perhaps because of technological change, so that few now try to dislodge you.

Positional advantage as a pecking order resonates with a wide variety of other social scientists, albeit from widely divergent value positions. Mauss (1970) studied the 'potlatch' feasts of the native American tribes, through which they strove to improve or at least protect their positions of honour. Veblen (1899) castigated the 'leisure class', whose conspicuous consumption advertised their success and reinforced their social and economic distance from the larger society. In the postwar period, many US sociologists portrayed their society as underpinned by a widely shared acceptance of just such a pecking order: an endorsement which served to legitimate prevailing inequalities (for a strong critique, see Goldthorpe and Hope (1972)).

In short: the one-dimensional view of positional advantage highlights the way that social actors strive for the best possible position in a pecking order. The latter involves a monotonic structuring of positions, which confer greater or lesser advantage and allow the occupant to dictate – or at least to influence – who else should be admitted or excluded. Growing prosperity has, however, turned this into an endless race, by opening to all the symbols of the pecking order such as education credentials and levels of consumption: as a result the levels required for any particular position are only inflated. As Hirsch says, 'the race gets longer for the same prize' (Hirsch, 1977: 67).

5.3 The two-dimensional view: positional advantage as connection across boundaries

The language of positional advantage is not merely that of 'more' and 'less', but also of access and exclusion. This is a language of incompletely connected positions. Not every position is connected to every other; and it is by standing astride particular connections that I can block your access, or ensure that you gain access only on my terms. Positional advantage here involves the establishing, maintaining and contesting not of a pecking order but of these connections across boundaries. This is no longer a monotonic ordering; and instead of trying to pass or leapfrog those above me in a pecking order, I can now build advantage by going round them. This we will refer to as the *two-dimensional view of positional advantage*.

Consider the military or naval commander preparing for battle. The general seeks to come at his enemy from high ground, the admiral from upwind. If he notices that his enemy has by-passed him and now commands the high ground or the upwind position, he knows he is in danger. So far this is akin to the one-dimensional positional advantage just discussed. However, the general seeks not only the high ground, but also the ground that allows easy transition to other strategic vantage points. A strategic vantage point is such, not only because it offers the high ground, but also because it allows easy access to a multitude of alternative vantage points from which to view the battlefield, see round corners, identify opportunities and threats and take action accordingly.[4]

Burt has based much of his sociological contribution upon such a notion of positional advantage. Thus, for example, he describes a 'structural hole' as a region across which there are no connections (Burt, 2004). Those who move to straddle such holes can then with advantage trade goods, services and ideas across the divide.

Burt explores the dynamics of such trade through various forms of network analysis. As in the one-dimensional case, a race can develop, as new bridges are built to straddle 'structural holes', and the positional advantages embedded in the geometry of connections are variously put in question. Towns that have grown up at the lowest bridging point of a river become back-waters, when advances in bridge-building technology allow a crossing point to be built downstream. Those whose positions are threatened may, however, resist: attempting to convert such potentially disruptive technologies into ones that sustain their own entrenched interests (Christensen, 2003).

Burt points to the wide variety of scholars, including Schumpeter, Simmel and Merton, who previously developed similar arguments. There are also connections with Granovetter's discussion of strong and weak ties (Granovetter, 1973): weak ties involve precisely the broker roles to which Burt appeals. Perri 6 (1996) then uses Granovetter to address social policy questions in new ways, in terms of the broker roles on which disadvantaged groups may be able to draw and the role of public policies in strengthening their weak ties.

Any structural hole may tend to close up, as rivals outflank the broker and enlarge the range of connections between communities hitherto separated. Here again, therefore, positional advantage may tend to dissipate. As with its one-dimensional counterpart, positional advantage has a past (in the sense of being shaped by yesterday's outcomes) and a future (in the sense of being forever at risk of dissipating).

Nevertheless, it is not only the bridging of boundaries that brings advantage: the latter can also arise from the maintenance of separation. Such separation can provide stability, protection against intrusive predation, the consolidation of a 'hinterland'. John Darwin (2007), in his account of European empire-building from the eighteenth century onwards, considers how different Asian countries were able to preserve an autonomous social, economic and political hinterland, as a basis for resilience and resistance, in face of European incursions. Which bridges are built, which hinterlands are protected, will affect different groups in different ways, and shape the positional advantages that they variously enjoy.

A similar analysis can be made of current struggles over the direction and degree of 'Europeanisation' within the EU and the maintenance of national policy autonomy, national social and economic spaces (Papadopoulos and Roumpakis, 2011). The geometry of these spaces will shape the positional advantage that different interest groups enjoy: it is therefore no surprise that this geometry is much contested. Much of the current drive for Europeanisation plays to corporate interests; a Europe where local communities drove the building of bridges and the development of 'weak ties' might be quite different (Room, 2007).

International alliances can also be understood in terms of such two-dimensional positional advantage. Jervis analyses how a State may be able to gain a pivotal position in relation to two others, by exploiting their entrenched conflict of interests and mutual hostility, so as to preserve its own freedom of manoeuvre. However, such a State may sometimes find that it is to its advantage to promote reconciliation of these two adversaries: for each of them, the friend of my friend should be my friend also. This is an analysis in terms of 'structural balance' within networks of connections (Jervis, 1997: chs 5–6).

In short, the two-dimensional view recognises that positions are incompletely connected with – and accessible to – each other: it is this very incompleteness that allows positional advantage to be enjoyed. The pursuit of positional advantage involves making new connections between hitherto unconnected positions, so as to exercise leverage over the social relations and social actors newly connected; or, alternatively, resisting those new connections in order to consolidate and retain existing advantage.

5.4 The three-dimensional view: positional advantage as command over dynamic synergies

The two-dimensional view depicts a landscape of incompletely connected positions. Positional advantage is sought and secured in terms of access, separation and exclusion across that landscape.

The social world is not, however, limited to a single landscape and struggle. Advantages won in one struggle can be mobilised in another: not only increasing the resources which the victors can deploy there, but also their scope for shaping the very rules of the game in that other arena (Lieberson, 1987).

Positional advantage, here, involves not the establishing, contesting and maintaining of a pecking order, nor indeed of connections across boundaries, but a race for the dynamic synergies across interrelated terrains that can endlessly reinforce and protect that advantage (see also Part I of this book). It also involves blocking the efforts of opponents to establish such dynamic synergies in relation to their own position.

This we refer to as the *three-dimensional view of positional advantage*. Positional advantage is now more than just an ascent within a given pecking order; and more than just the extraction of advantage from the connections across an incompletely connected world. It is command and control of the positive feedback processes and dynamic synergies that will shape future pecking orders and connective advantages. This perspective is what previous chapters have referred to as transformative realism.

Such a view of positional advantage is evident in the work of Pierson (2004). In his account of institutional dynamics, he gives considerable importance to 'first mover advantage': in other words, to whichever actor first occupies a particular institutional terrain. Such occupation can set positive feedback processes in motion, which reinforce the position of the first occupier and define the setting to which losers have then to accommodate themselves. Potts makes a parallel argument in relation to entrepreneurs and their innovations (Potts, 2000). Nevertheless, there is forever the haunting fear that others will steal an innovative march; it is this above all that keeps first movers on their mettle (Dopfer and Potts, 2008: para. 4.2.1). Both Pierson and Potts highlight the ways in which first movers will, therefore, typically institute further waves of innovation and can often do so rather effectively, from the position of strength they have won. This can produce a 'winner-take-all' society (Hacker and Pierson, 2010).

A similar account of the struggle for positional advantage was central to papers published by Goldthorpe from the mid-1970s onwards, concerned with the political economy of western industrial societies, after the post-war decades of economic expansion (Goldthorpe, 1974, 1978, 1984, 1985). Faltering growth confronted policy-makers with a zero-sum distributional game, to an extent which until then had been avoidable. The welfare 'settlements' of the post-war period now came under intense strain, as organised labour and capital each sought to escape the zero-sum game and avoid positional disadvantage. These struggles ranged beyond the realm of welfare policy narrowly conceived: from education to the labour market, to the social security system and the housing market. Advantage gained on one terrain shifted the balance of forces available to contest another, outflanking established institutional arrangements and forging new opportunities for leverage.

The race for such positional advantage can tend to reinforce uncertainty and insecurity: producing what Hobbes described as the 'war of each against all', Durkheim as the *anomie* of capitalist societies. It is a struggle to ensure that come what may, tomorrow will turn out well for the protagonists in question, allowing them to weave their own destinies, rather than being obliged to move to the rhythms of others (Abbott, 2001: 247). Social actors strive for positional advantage so as to maintain their freedom of manoeuvre, keeping others guessing as to what they will do next; to block developments they oppose; to offload uncertainty onto others and destabilise them, so that they are locked into a minimal set of possible strategies and cannot mount a challenge (Marris, 1996; Pierson, 2004). This is why, as Keynes for example observes, the accumulation of wealth is often not so much for eventual consumption, it is for some indefinitely distant date, to ensure a place in the sun, whatever the future disposition of the world (Tily, 2007: 142). It is in this sense that the three-dimensional view depicts positional advantage as a struggle *to design and occupy the future.*

In short: the three-dimensional view recognises that positions provide opportunities to reshape a wider range of connections, thereby exploiting dynamic synergies that can turn advantage into further advantage. The consequences may, however, be difficult to foresee, and they may involve dramatic reconfigurations of social arrangements. The struggle for positional advantage is thus a struggle to offload uncertainty onto others and to build resilience and a protected vantage point, whatever the future.

5.5 Positional advantage as occupation

Positional advantage involves the *occupation* of a position. The one-dimensional view of positional advantage involves occupation of the high ground, in a monotonic ordering. The two-dimensional view involves occupation of space and the connections between spaces. The three-dimensional view involves 'occupation of the future', offloading onto others the uncertainties which the future unavoidably entails, and mobilising the transformative dynamics that can capture and reinforce that occupation.

At the start of this chapter, this discussion of positions was located within the literature on social stratification. By occupying a particular position, someone enjoys status, political power and material benefits and they can exclude others from them. Occupancy thus involves some security of tenure. It may thereby also grant 'rents' on scarce assets or through intellectual property rights on innovations long past (see also Chapter 9 below).

Occupancy offers the 'settled ground' of knowledge and conventional practices from which social actors 'probe' the uncertain and foggy landscapes on which they find themselves: see our discussion of 'agile action' in Chapter 4.

We are concerned, therefore, not just with a position within a system of stratification, but also with the adaptive walks that are possible from this vantage point, involving changes in the resources and capabilities of the actors themselves. This is what Abbott (Abbott, 2001: ch. 5) captures in his discussion of interdependent 'careers': whether applied to individuals, professions or communities.

Finally, let us notice that a position may be invaded and occupied by others, with a view to exploiting its advantages or denying them to others. The most obvious case is the military occupation of a territory and the subjugation of its population. This forces them to dance to the invader's tune, as the invaders impose their own settled understanding and practices: albeit some may find that tune not uncongenial, and a means of enhancing their own positions. Darwin (2007), as we have seen, recounts how different Asian countries varied in their resilience and resistance, in face of the European incursions: even so, there were plenty of local actors who found a niche in the European imperia. Deák recounts similarly how, under German occupation during the Second World War, the countries of Europe saw different groups of social actors responding quite differently to the threats – but also the opportunities – that occupation brought: and had afterwards to live with the tangled social divisions which the occupation thus bequeathed (Deák et al., 2000).

5.6 Positional advantage and power

At the outset to this chapter, we recognised that any treatment of positional advantage – the focus of this chapter – would inevitably have implications for debates on power. It is to these that we now turn.

Weber is commonly taken as the starting point for sociological discussions of power. He famously defined power in terms of an actor's capacity to enforce his or her will, even in face of the resistance and opposition of others (Gerth and Mills, 1948: ch. 7). One aspect of power – which Weber perhaps fails to stress – is that not only can you get your way, despite the possible resistance of others, but that you can do so *at a time of your choosing*. The fewer the moments – and the more limited the circumstances – that their resistance can withstand you, the greater can your power be said to be, the fewer the contingencies under which it is frustrated. The absence of such resistance does not, however, mean that power is not being exercised: the simple *threat* of exercising it may be sufficient to deter resistance.

Weber focuses our attention on agency, will, capacity and resistance and on the institutional context within which power is possessed and exercised. The same goes for the discussion by Goldthorpe and Bevan with which the present chapter started. For them, unequal advantage is manifested in structures of hierarchical differentiation, underpinned by institutional arrangements, and power is the capacity to secure such advantage. 'Advantage' is a distributional aspect of stratification, while 'power' is the relational counterpart.

Building on Weber, we might then define power as the capacity of an actor to secure positional advantage, in given social and institutional conditions, even in face of the resistance and opposition of others. This resonates also with Lukes (2005), the other major point of reference for recent debates on power, in particular through our discussion of three 'dimensions' of positional advantage.[5]

Lukes starts from the assumption, made by American political scientists such as Dahl (1957), that power within democratic political institutions is wielded by voting strength within deliberative assemblies. This is what Lukes describes as the first dimension of power. It is the pecking order of those who control these votes.

Against this, he sets the power to shape and limit what issues get onto the voting agenda at all. This is his second dimension of power. More generally it is about powerful actors being able to shape, re-mould, sort and select, from among the items that *might* in principle get onto the agenda. In other words, it is about access and exclusion.

Finally, Lukes appeals to such writers as Gramsci, to argue that the cultural power of particular social groups may be such as to hide from the disadvantaged the way that their interests and needs are systematically disregarded. It is around the conceptual definition of this third dimension of power, and its empirical investigation, that much of the subsequent debate with Lukes has centred.[6]

As one of his principal illustrations of this third dimension, Lukes takes the cultural power of the Catholic Church, in shaping the perceptions and aspirations of the poor. This may seem to have little connection with our own third dimension of positional advantage, as a race for dynamic synergies. Instead it centres in the cultural stasis that the Church is able to impose. Nevertheless, the empirical evidence that this stasis is indeed imposed, and that power is being actively exercised to this end, requires that we point to a counterfactual: of similar communities that have thrown off such alleged constraints and are articulating their 'true' needs, albeit with a struggle. This is central to the methodological inferences that Lukes draws from his conceptual argument.

Gaventa (who developed his doctoral research under Lukes) applied these ideas to mining communities in the Appalachians, comparing them, but also considering how they changed over time (Gaventa, 1980). Room similarly applied Lukes to community action projects within the European anti-poverty programmes (Room, 1986: ch. 4). This study examined and compared how these communities could, through action-research initiatives, develop a quite different and more critical perspective from the one with which each of them started.

Thus both Gaventa and Room use Lukes' third dimension of power to understand the processes of change and self-enlightenment within such communities, as they contested the dominant assumptions of the larger political and economic order within which they found themselves. Both writers seek to capture the dynamic and endogenous processes of change under way in these communities, as the people concerned uncovered the connections between the advantages of the powerful and the living conditions of their own communities. By questioning the dominant wisdom and levering change, these communities strove, to some degree, to build resilience for the future. It is to just such dynamic processes that our three-dimensional discussion of positional advantage has pointed.

5.7 Positional advantage and fitness landscapes

The three-dimensional view of positional advantage is framed in terms of a race for the dynamic synergies across interrelated terrains that can endlessly reinforce and protect that advantage. Such a race for dynamic synergies has also been central to evolutionary models of change and, more particularly, to processes of co-evolution. Our account of positional advantage, therefore, also impinges on the vexed debates as to how evolutionary perspectives can most appropriately be applied to the social world (see also Chapter 2 above). It is to the value of such evolutionary models in the analysis of positional advantage that we finally turn.

Biological evolution is a 'blind' process, without overall intent or purpose, which selects those 'variations' or sub-species which are best adapted to the abiotic and biotic environment in question. This is biological 'fitness', although even here it is not altogether straightforward to define such fitness, nor indeed to predict in advance which variants will excel in a given environment.

One of the iconic metaphors of such evolution is of an 'adaptive walk' across a 'fitness landscape', which may be more or less rugged (Figure 5.1).[7] Each species can be thought of as occupying such a landscape. Under pressure from the 'struggle for existence', through minor genetic mutations (changes in the horizontal coordinates) it ascends the hillside and increases its fitness. Of course, this notion of an 'adaptive walk' is to some degree a fiction, inasmuch as the 'walk' is undertaken blind, and not by individuals but by populations over the course of many generations, as one or other of these mutations proves differentially able to thrive within this particular environment. Nevertheless, the fiction can be illuminating and convenient.

No species makes its evolutionary journey in isolation. For species such as insects and flowering plants, although far removed from each other in the evolutionary 'Tree of Life', the contours of their fitness landscapes are dynamically linked. As one species makes its adaptive walk across its fitness landscape, the consequent changes in its phenotype will modify the adaptive landscape on which the other finds itself. It is the discovery and exploitation of such mutual benefits that has produced the wonderful adaptations to each other that our flora and fauna exhibit. The evolutionary journey of a species is thus

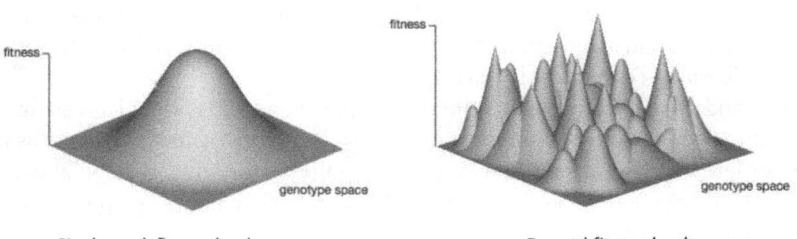

Single peak fitness landscape   Rugged fitness landscape

Figure 5.1 Fitness landscapes

104 *Agile actors*

path-dependent by reference not only to its own genetic legacy (the point on the fitness landscape at which it started), but also to the ecosystems of which it has become part. It is on the contingent combination of this dual legacy that natural selection acts.[8]

When we apply evolutionary models to the social world, it is with a view to illuminating a similar dynamic. At first glance there is a straightforward parallel. Human creativity continuously throws up myriad innovations in the technological and institutional forms with which social actors deal. These are variously taken up by the wider population, with some becoming dominant across the society at large. Evolutionary economists analyse markets as examples of such selection mechanisms (Beinhocker, 2007; Dopfer and Potts, 2008; Hodgson and Knudsen, 2010). Political scientists likewise analyse the social and political processes by which particular institutional innovations are selected (Pierson, 2004; Crouch, 2005; Streek and Thelen, 2005).

Nevertheless, it is not sufficient to treat such selection mechanisms as 'blind' forms of 'self-organisation'. Powerful actors struggle purposefully to organise and reshape these processes and the direction of technological and institutional change, so as to reinforce and defend their own positional advantage. Here there is an endless dance, between the purposeful efforts of social actors, to shape the overall dynamics of a society in pursuit of their positional advantage, and the myriad processes of micro-innovation and selection which blindly self-organise (for a more extended treatment, see Chapters 2 and 3 above) (Room, 2012).

What do we mean by 'fitness' in relation to social dynamics? It means in part the satisfaction of the consumer in the market place. It means also what powerful actors reckon will favour their interests and their positional advantage. 'Fitness' here is something that human innovators attempt to judge *ex ante*, rather than just waiting for it to be revealed *ex post*. Indeed, 'fitness' here gives way to 'positional advantage' as the most appropriate organising concept for understanding such selection processes.

From this vantage point, the foregoing perspectives on fitness landscapes can be used to depict the strategic environment within which social actors find themselves, as they struggle for positional advantage. Here they take stock of the path dependencies of their past investments; and here they experiment with new combinations of technologies and institutions, in hope of discovering new co-evolutionary synergies. This involves selective probing, trying out imaginative new combinations and discovering their potential, not randomly but by systematic testing and learning (Bronowski, 1981: chs 2–4).

Fitness landscapes neatly capture our three dimensions of positional advantage. Our first dimension was a one-dimensional metric, with positional advantage as a pecking order. Our landscape likewise presents fitness – or now, in a social context, positional advantage – as the height of the landscape at any given point. This is a one-dimensional metric.

However, we can also study the shape of different landscapes of positional advantage and the ease of strategic journeys to higher points. Compare the smooth and single-peaked landscape in Figure 5.1 with the rugged landscape. In the former, whatever the starting point, a strategic walk towards higher ground is readily accomplished through successive small steps. The rugged landscape, in contrast, offers a world of incompletely connected positions: it is easy to get stuck on a low peak, from which ascents to greater fitness are blocked by deep valleys. These constitute what, following Burt, we referred to as 'structural holes', when we presented positional advantage as two-dimensional. It is only by bridging such holes – discovering ridges that span deep valleys – that fitness (now reconceptualised as positional advantage) can be enhanced.

The dynamics of inter-linked landscapes, central to accounts of co-evolution, are also central to our third dimension of positional advantage. Students of biological evolution have identified the variety of forms that such dynamics can take. Some may settle into an 'evolutionarily stable state' of mutual adjustment (the evolutionary analogue of a Nash equilibrium in game theory) (Maynard Smith, 1982). However, they may also take the form of a 'Red Queen', a race in which each co-evolving species produces turmoil in the fitness landscapes of the others. These dynamics have been fruitfully applied by evolutionary economists (Dopfer and Potts, 2008).

These contested processes have to be understood by reference to the political economy of the societies in question. Much of the social science literature that applies evolutionary perspectives to social change fails to give any central place to power and advantage: core concepts within any sociological account of social differentiation and social order. This is not perhaps surprising among those who retain a focus on the biological substrate of human behaviour (for example, Sloan Wilson, 2008); but even among those who explicitly abandon that biological legacy (for example, Dopfer and Potts, 2008), an explicit engagement with power and politics is rare. In opposition to this neglect, we bring the exercise of power centre-stage, in any attempt to apply evolutionary models to the social world. It is by reference to our three-dimensional analysis of the struggle for positional advantage that this can most readily be done.

5.8 Conclusion

Our starting point was the influential account of positional advantage offered by Hirsch (1977). Hirsch's purpose was, however, not limited to a conceptual illumination of 'positional advantage'. He wanted to diagnose the 'social limits to growth' that this struggle entailed and to lay out the implications for public policy. It is with these implications for policy debate that this chapter therefore concludes.

First, Hirsch argues that the positional competition at the heart of affluent societies is wasteful and self-defeating. Possessive individualism has played a key role in the culture of industrialisation but it is now a hindrance. What is needed instead is collective action to moderate the race and to spread more evenly the benefits of a highly productive economy. In Keynes' words, the game should be played for lower stakes. Otherwise the winner-take-all society will be an arena of corrosive *anomie*: not 'Smithian harmony' but 'Hobbesian strife' (Hirsch, 1977: ch. 13).

The four decades that have passed since Hirsch's book appeared have seen public provision and collective action in retreat across the affluent world. Hirsch bemoans the 'depleting moral legacy' which could support the collective action for which he calls: since he wrote, it has been depleted all the more. Meanwhile concerns about environmental damage have underlined the case for collective action – and the calamity that political failure to moderate the positional competition is liable to produce.

Our three-dimensional account of the struggle for positional advantage strengthens Hirsch's analysis. The positional competition is not limited to the inflation of educational credentials and the cultural symbols of the leisure class. It involves a struggle that can undermine modes of living and sow radical uncertainty and insecurity. The corollary for public policy is that government can and should provide an environment of greater certainty and resilience for citizens, in which they can make longer-term decisions and investments, and make their creative contributions to society. This is consistent with the account of agile action we developed in Chapter 4. This contrasts however with the policy rhetoric of consumer choice and behaviour change, which have dominated discussion in recent years, rooted in a quite different understanding of social action.

The race for ever-higher levels of personal consumption is arguably less about meeting our needs, more about social inclusion and a sense of security. However, growing inequality within rich societies only reinforces the race to keep up with unsustainable lifestyles and our 'inertia' in face of government pleas that we change our behaviour. Emulation of those lifestyles by the new middle classes of the emerging economies means globalisation of that insecurity.

Central to this insecurity is the cultural and economic power of the super-rich – what Veblen (1899) described as the 'leisure class' – with their conspicuous consumption and their selective recruitment of the new rich of the emerging economies. They alone have flourished during the present austerity (see, for example, Congressional Budget Office, 2013). Piketty (2014) warns that growing inequality will be a feature of the twenty-first century and will undermine democratic values.

Therefore, what may be needed – and this is very much in the spirit of Hirsch's own book – is a sober national debate, as to how our resources and capacities can be harnessed to address environmental sustainability, and a new social contract providing security for all within creative communities. Within such communities, it may be possible to develop new social practices of collective responsibility for our shared future: building institutions that educate in civility and civic concern and which 'emphasise and strengthen, not the class differences which divide, but the common humanity that unites' us (Tawney, 1931, 1964: 49). It may then be politically feasible to move towards equitable and sustainable lifestyles, where we are all content with less. But this presupposes a radical attack on inequality.

These are all policy issues that will be examined at greater length in Part III of this book.

Notes

1 The distinction between 'material' and 'positional' goods was not original to Hirsch: a similar distinction is, for example, made in Keynes' essay, 'Economic Possibilities for our Grandchildren' (1952).
2 In regards to education, Brown and Lauder have recently updated and reinforced Hirsch's conceptual and empirical argument (Brown *et al.*, 2011).
3 In the 2012 Olympics, competitors in the 100- and 200-metre sprint events commented that they took for granted that Bolt would win the gold, so they left him to get on with it, and concentrated on the competition for the silver and bronze. This situation is also well-recognised in game theory. A Stackelberg game is a sequential game, but limited to a single round: one player goes first and others have then to accommodate themselves as best they can, on the terrain the first mover has already occupied (Stackelberg, 1952; Tirole, 1988: 8.2). Stackelberg applied this to industries with a dominant firm. He depicts a nested structure of positional advantage within the resulting market: 'The oligopolists of the first category rule the roost and they fight for the most favourable positions in the market. The oligopolists of the second category must adjust their position to that of the stronger competitors, but they compete with one another for the crumbs left by the latter. [Similarly], those of the third category take their cue from the first and second categories and help to dominate the next categories below them.' As Stackelberg notes, such a market enjoys greater stability than simple oligopoly because there are clear distinctions in terms of size and power. Similar pecking orders are common among communities of predators.
4 The Oxford philosopher J.L.H. Thomas has pointed out that many philosophical categories can be seen as expressions of the distinction between past, present and future. What is the spatial counterpart of these temporal distinctions? Thomas responds in terms of here, there and 'otherwhere' (personal communication). Otherwhere is a place which is accessible from 'there' but not from 'here'. Positional advantage involves command over access to otherwhere.
5 Lukes has nuanced his original argument in a number of ways, in response to the critics, but has retained the core of his original argument (see, for example, the 2006 *Political Studies Review* symposium and the response that Lukes (2006) makes there to his critics).
6 It was with his third dimension that Lukes rested his case. Subsequent writers such as Foucault and Bourdieu have developed broader accounts of power in capitalist societies. See Lukes (2005: 89–107, 139–43) for his own assessment of both, in relation to these conceptual and methodological debates.
7 Recent exponents of fitness landscapes include Kauffman (1993, 1995) and Gavrilets (2004). The origins of the metaphor are to be found in Fisher (1930) and Wright (1932).
8 The classic discussion of contingency in evolution is Gould (1991: chs IV–V).

References

Abbott, A. (2001), *Time Matters: On Theory and Method*, Chicago, IL: University of Chicago Press
Beinhocker, E.D. (2007), *The Origin of Wealth*, London: Random House
Bronowski, J. (1981), *The Ascent of Man*, London: Futura
Brown, P., H. Lauder, and D. Ashton (2011), *The Global Auction*, Oxford: Oxford University Press
Burt, R.S. (2004), 'Structural Holes and Good Ideas', *American Journal of Sociology*, 110(2): 349–99
Christensen, C.M. (2003), *The Innovator's Dilemma*, New York: HarperCollins

Congressional Budget Office (2013), *The Distribution of Household Income and Federal Taxes, 2010,* Washington, DC: Congress of the United States

Crouch, C. (2005), *Capitalist Diversity and Change: Recombinant Governance and Institutional Entrepreneurs,* Oxford: Oxford University Press

Dahl, R.A. (1957), 'The Concept of Power', *Behavioural Science,* 2: 201–5

Darwin, J. (2007), *After Tamerlane: The Rise and Fall of Global Empires, 1400–2000,* Harmondsworth: Penguin

Dawe, A. (1970), 'The Two Sociologies', *British Journal of Sociology,* 21(2): 207–18

Deák, I., J.T. Gross, and T. Judt, (eds) (2000), *The Politics of Retribution in Europe,* Princeton, NJ: Princeton University Press

Dopfer, K. and J. Potts (2008), *The General Theory of Economic Evolution,* London: Routledge

Fisher, R.A. (1930), *The Genetical Theory of Natural Selection,* Oxford: Clarendon Press

Gaventa, J. (1980), *Power and Powerlessness: Quiescence and Rebellion in an Appalachian Valley,* Oxford: Clarendon Press

Gavrilets, S. (2004), *Fitness Landscapes and the Origin of Species,* Princeton, NJ: Princeton University Press

Gerth, H.H. and C.W. Mills (1948), *From Max Weber: Essays in Sociology,* London: Routledge

Goldthorpe, J.H. (1974), 'Social Inequality and Social Integration in Modern Britain', in D. Wedderburn (ed.), *Poverty, Inequality and Class Structure,* Cambridge: Cambridge University Press: 217–34

Goldthorpe, J.H. (1978), 'The Current Inflation: Towards a Sociological Account', in F. Hirsch and J. H. Goldthorpe (eds), *The Political Economy of Inflation,* London: Martin Robertson: 186–216

Goldthorpe, J.H. (1984), *Order and Conflict in Contemporary Capitalism,* Oxford: Oxford University Press

Goldthorpe, J.H. (1985), 'Problems of Political Economy after the End of the Post-War Period', in C. S. Maier (ed.), *Changing Boundaries of the Political,* Oxford: Oxford University Press: 363–407

Goldthorpe, J.H. and P. Bevan (1977), 'The Study of Social Stratification in Great Britain 1945–75', *Social Science Information,* 16(3–4): 279–334

Goldthorpe, J.H. and K. Hope (1972), 'Occupational Grading and Occupational Prestige', in K. Hope (ed.), *The Analysis of Social Mobility,* Oxford: Clarendon Press

Gould, S.J. (1991), *Wonderful Life,* Harmondsworth: Penguin

Granovetter, M. (1973), 'The Strength of Weak Ties', *American Journal of Sociology,* 78: 1360–80

Hacker, J.S. and P. Pierson (2010), *Winner-Take-All Politics,* New York: Simon and Schuster

Hirsch, F. (1977), *Social Limits to Growth,* London: Routledge and Kegan Paul

Hodgson, G.M. and T. Knudsen (2010), *Darwin's Conjecture: The Search for General Principles of Social and Economic Evolution,* Chicago, IL: University of Chicago Press

Jervis, R. (1997), *System Effects: Complexity in Political and Social Life,* Princeton, NJ: Princeton University Press

Kauffman, S.A. (1993), *The Origins of Order: Self-Organisation and Selection in Evolution,* Oxford: Oxford University Press

Kauffman, S.A. (1995), *At Home in the Universe: The Search for Laws of Self-Organisation and Complexity,* Harmondsworth: Penguin

Keynes, J.M. (1952), *Essays in Persuasion*, London: Hart-Davies
Lieberson, S. (1987), *Making it Count: The Improvement of Social Research and Theory*, Berkeley: University of California Press
Lukes, S.M. (2005), *Power: A Radical View (Second Edition)*, Basingstoke: Palgrave Macmillan
Lukes, S.M. (2006), 'Reply to Comments', *Political Studies Review*, 4(2): 164–73
Marris, P. (1996), *The Politics of Uncertainty*, London: Routledge
Mauss, M. (1970), *The Gift*, London: Routledge and Kegan Paul
Maynard Smith, J. (1982), *Evolution and the Theory of Games*, Cambridge: Cambridge University Press
Papadopoulos, T. and A. Roumpakis (2011), 'Nordic Social Risk Management and the Challenge of EU Regulation: Labour Market Parity at Risk', in V.-P. Sorsa (ed.), *Rethinking Social Risk in the Nordics*, Foundation of European Progressive Studies: 199–224
Perri 6 (1996), *Escaping Poverty*, London: Demos
Pierson, P. (2004), *Politics in Time*, Princeton, NJ: Princeton University Press
Piketty, T. (2014), *Capital in the Twenty-First Century*, Cambridge, MA: Belknap/Harvard University Press
Potts, J. (2000), *The New Evolutionary Microeconomics: Complexity, Competence and Adaptive Behaviour*, Cheltenham: Edward Elgar
Room, G. (1986), *Cross-National Innovation in Social Policy*, London: Macmillan
Room, G. (2007), 'Challenges Facing the EU: Scope for a Coherent Response', *European Societies*, 9(3): 229–44
Room, G. (2012), 'Evolution and the Arts of Civilisation', *Policy and Politics*, 40(4): 453–71
Sloan Wilson, D. (2008), 'Multilevel Selection Theory and Major Evolutionary Transitions', *Current Directions in Psychological Science*, 17(1): 6–9
Stackelberg, H.v. (1952), *The Theory of the Market Economy (Grundlage der Theoretischen Volkswirtschaftslehre, 1948: translated with an Introduction by Alan T Peacock)*, London: William Hodge
Streek, W. and K. Thelen, (eds) (2005), *Beyond Continuity: Institutional Change in Advanced Political Economies*, Oxford: Oxford University Press
Tawney, R.H. (1931, 1964), *Equality*, London: Unwin Books
Tily, G. (2007), *Keynes's General Theory, The Rate of Interest and 'Keynesian' Economics: Keynes Betrayed*, London: Palgrave Macmillan
Tirole, J. (1988), *The Theory of Industrial Organization*, Cambridge, MA: The MIT Press
Veblen, T. (1899), *The Theory of the Leisure Class*, New York: Macmillan
Wright, S. (1932), 'The Roles of Mutation, Inbreeding, Crossbreeding and Selection in Evolution', in D.F. Jones (ed.), *Proceedings of the Sixth International Congress on Genetics*, 1: 356–66

6 Navigating complex environments

6.1 Introduction

In a complex and evolving social and economic 'ecosystem', individual actors face uncertainty as to how the future will unfold, and what consequences will follow from any train of action that they pursue. Nevertheless, the majority of our actions each day involve 'ordinary' situations which we handle almost unthinkingly, using standard templates and rules of thumb. These we learn as members of society, adapting them to our own particular contexts. This is what Weber (1949: ch. 2) described as 'habitual' action.

Here is some solid ground: an expanse that is safe and predictable: a vantage point that involves a settled body of knowledge and practices. Of course, even these are never wholly secure in face of adversity or unexpected bounty. Redundancy at work, bereavement or a disaster such as an earthquake or a tsunami can disrupt the meaning and coherence that habitual routines provide and incapacitate those concerned. So can sudden wealth.[1]

The realm of the habitual is readily handled by standard rules of thumb: these leave social actors free to devote most of their attention to novel problems and to probe terrains as yet unexplored. They deploy mental models as to how the world is likely to unfold and how they may be able to steer and shape it. This is all the more demanding when they are faced with fellow actors who are also seeking to steer it, but in quite different directions.

This is 'agile' action (see Chapter 4 above). It is when actors detect anomalous patterns (including, for example, those that fall outside certain critical thresholds) that they are alerted to the need for a response which does not rely on the standard templates of the habitual. These are situations that may present opportunities or threats of major existential significance for the actors in question. Which matters are handled in which way is itself therefore fluid; and this will vary between actors, depending on their interests and the resources and positional leverage of which they dispose.

This chapter is concerned with how social actors 'read' such complex terrains in real time, instead of just extrapolating from the accumulated evidence of past experience. They use simple heuristics to detect impending threats or opportunities: these are discussed in terms of thresholds, alignments and sequences.

In acting, they use mental models of how the world is likely to unfold. Such actions take time to work through: the actors involved, therefore, require real-time information as to how things are changing: they must have some way of evaluating this and drawing appropriate lessons. The chapter concludes with the implications for empirical research and for policy advice.

Some of the illustrations used will be taken from sailing and navigation at sea: including 'reading' the sea and the weather conditions.[2] The same metaphor is used by a variety of other writers who sail these particular waters: see for example Scott (1998: ch. 9). But of course, any such illustration has its limitations, and we must be careful when applying these to the social and policy worlds, lest we drown in misplaced analogies. Not least, to read the sea and the weather – and other natural phenomena – involves no reading of intentions: those of a strategic opponent, for example, part of whose skill may lie precisely in concealing those intentions (Jervis, 1997: 44–8, 253–8).[3]

6.2 Bounded rationality

'Agile' action goes beyond rational action theory as normally articulated (see also Chapter 4 above). There, the social actor is confronted with a given menu of options, carrying particular costs, benefits and consequences, whose overall utility he or she calculates. Here, however, the agile actor, rather than taking that menu as given, actively reshapes the institutional and technological landscape on which social interactions play out, precisely so as to reshape the options it offers.

There is a considerable if varied literature on 'bounded rationality', which recognises that the orthodox treatment of the rational actor suffers from a number of limitations. Some is strongly influenced by the 'complexity' perspectives on which the present book draws. It is therefore worth considering the affinities and contrasts with our own account of agile action.

First, social actors have incomplete information, not least in regards to the future. Rational expectations theory responds by assuming that the actor nevertheless knows the range of possible outcomes or futures and the probability of each (Simon, 1969: ch. 2). Appropriately nuanced, much of the orthodox treatment of the rational actor can be retained. More problematic is if we recognise that some outcomes or futures are *uncertain*. Uncertainty differs from risk inasmuch as no probabilities can be pre-assigned to the various possible outcomes. Matters are worse still if even the range of possible outcomes cannot be delimited with any confidence.

The second version of 'bounded rationality' refers to the cognitive limitations of individual actors: the limits of their ability to reason logically, in relation to the choices that they face. Kahneman (2011), for example, distinguishes between 'fast' and 'slow' thinking. The former involves simple rules of thumb ('heuristics'), the latter more considered and systematic assessment of a situation. Most of our actions – if only because of the hectic multiplicity of situations we face in any one day – are addressed by fast thinking. This distinction between 'fast' and 'slow' thinking may therefore appear similar to that between habitual and agile action, as elaborated above (see also Chapter 4).

Behaviourists such as Thaler and Sunstein (2009) argue that the rules of thumb embodied in 'fast' thinking tend to produce decisions replete with biases and blunders.[4] This is quite different from the settled body of knowledge and practices that we have associated with habitual action. Moreover, we treat habits and rules of thumb not as psychological traits, but as residues of collective learning, carried in communities and institutions and shaped by the social, political and economic order. This does not imply that those habits and rules of thumb are unproblematic. The understandings and practices with which people operate may produce consequences which, under interrogation, they may disavow and for which they might not wish to be held accountable (see also Chapter 4 above). This sort of blunder and bias may extend from the 'least sophisticated' sections of the population, with which Thaler and Sunstein are primarily concerned, to elements of the sophisticated financial elite involved in the financial crisis of 2008 (see Chapters 8 and 9 below).

A third form of 'bounded rationality' follows from the inability of social actors, in complex environments, to anticipate the non-linear, dynamic and sometimes counter-intuitive consequences of their actions (Kauffman, 2008: ch. 14). The Schelling model of the emergence of racial segregation – an outcome unintended by any of those involved – provides a simple illustration (see Chapter 1 above). As noted earlier, this may be compounded by their limited ability to read and anticipate the intentions of others (Jervis, 1997).

It is in light of these limitations that we offer the notion of agile action. Here the actor keeps one foot on firm and stable ground, while investigating uncertain ground with the other, in a search for enhanced positional advantage (see also Chapters 4 and 5 above).

6.3 Agile probing for positional advantage

Agile actors stand on the stable vantage point of settled knowledge and practices. From here they can probe the world around them, notwithstanding the limitations of the information available and of their own cognitive processes. If, however, this safe and solid ground is too limited, they may have to hunker down, unable to venture further.

To probe is to move across the social landscape. This is a journey across a 'non-integral space', where not every point or space is connected to every other (Potts, 2000). This is, for example, central to Burt's account of 'structural holes' within the social networks in which social actors are embedded (Burt, 2004). Social actors must, therefore, find appropriate 'stepping stones' across which they can make their way: a task made all the more difficult if the walk must be accomplished in foggy conditions of incomplete information, and with the cognitive limitations just mentioned.[5] Here the social actor is not just calculating the utility of different choices and fashioning means to ends: he or she is moving so as to build positional advantage (see Chapter 5 above).

One way of modelling such walks is in terms of a Bayesian search and decision process. This involves developing hunches on the basis of settled knowledge. We accept provisionally the least bad explanation currently on offer and then see how far our empirical experience tends to support or undermine that explanation. This, however, is a path-dependent process, which we may only much later discover is misguided.[6]

The dynamics of such walks can also be explored in terms of a 'fitness landscape'. This is a tool developed originally in models of evolution by natural selection, but in principle it is applicable also to the purposive walks of agile social actors (see also Chapters 2 and 5 above). Here is a language for examining what walks are possible without the need for costly new investments in additional capacities (descents into valleys); the extent to which landscapes are dynamically interdependent; and the scope for predicting from a local terrain the contours of a wider expanse.[7]

However, to probe is to do more than walk across a landscape. These are 'adaptive walks', which also involve the opportunistic reshaping of the social landscape. Agile actors may seek to change the connective geometry of this landscape, switching and modifying the connections among its sub-systems (Simon, 1969: ch. 8; Stewart, 2001). They may try to mobilise its dynamic synergies, its generative mechanisms and non-linear dynamics, so as to discover new openings of which they can make use (see Chapter 1 above). Each step in this endeavour may involve them in drawing selectively on the *bricolage* of other endeavours, recycling this to their new ends. Even so, it is also quite possible that given their starting point, and the settled knowledge and practices from which they began, they remain confined in a *cul-de-sac*.

Social actors deploy mental models as to how the world is likely to unfold and how they can steer and shape it. A Bayesian hunch or a fitness landscape is just such a mental model. So is a Popperian theory (see Chapter 4 above). So is the chart that a mariner uses to navigate (notwithstanding that some – relying still on Admiralty surveys of the nineteenth century – may be little better than hunches). This means that while adaptive walks on uncertain terrains are generally made in small steps, this is not always the case. Social actors can employ mental models in order, to some degree, to imagine their world from other vantage points and to spot opportunities and dangers that are likely to emerge. These mental models may thus permit not just small steps but long jumps also (Kauffman, 1993: ch. 3; Jervis, 1997: 39).

They may also lead onto the rocks. Social actors will have built their portfolio of mental models and practices within the succession of niches which they have occupied, individually and collectively, and the insights but also the blind spots which each of these bequeathed. It is by understanding those careers that we can make sense of the mental models they bring to novel situations and the templates with which they operate.

In face of turbulence and uncertainty, agile actors will need to acquire new heuristics and mental models. To do this they must interrogate – and learn from – their neighbours and from actors with experience of other times and places.

This is a logic of cooperation and communication, a system of distributed intelligence (Christakis and Fowler, 2009). Eppel and Wolf argue for 'open, flexible access to multiple sources of expertise' (Eppel *et al.*, 2011: 184). Referring to the work of Jane Jacobs, Scott writes that 'complex, diverse, animated environments contribute ... to producing a resilient, flexible, adept population that has more experience in confronting novel challenges and taking initiative' (Scott, 1998: 349).

Neighbours differ greatly in their size, power and interests. Big actors can provide both stability and windows of opportunity; they can also provide connections to additional resources that would otherwise be too remote: connections that span 'small worlds' (Watts, 2003: ch. 3). Probing in the shadow of big actors can thus serve as a shortcut to a larger universe. However, it can also mean incorporation into their domains on adverse terms.

Such incorporation is not always in the best interests of the big actor itself. Christensen (2003: ch. 9) points out the difficulty that established industrial players find in developing innovations which lead in new directions ('disruptive technologies') rather than simply aligning with existing investments ('sustaining technologies'). They will typically need to establish a protected arena or hinterland, within which the potential of these innovations can be explored without regard to the settled ground of existing products. In general, it is only if they do this that established industrial players can probe new possibilities and progressively shift to new markets and value chains.

Finally, to probe the social world is to contest the meanings and claims that this world embodies: not just claims as to what is, but also claims as to what should be: including the entitlements and obligations which social actors have to each other and the hopes that they entertain.

6.4 Thresholds, alignments and sequences

Here we suggest three heuristics that are commonly employed to navigate complex and turbulent environments: and, more particularly, to recognise anomalous patterns for which a habit-based response based on settled patterns will not suffice, because they signal opportunities or threats of major potential significance for the actors in question.[8]

First, there may be a *threshold* whose crossing will bestir us to action. Goldthorpe, for example, in his modelling of social mobility, reckons that households are generally averse to downward mobility for their offspring: any signs that this threshold could be violated will tend to bring energetic counter-action by the parents (Goldthorpe, 2000: ch. 11). Schelling's model of racial segregation posits residents who must have at least a certain minimum proportion of their immediate neighbours drawn from the same ethnic group, if they are not to move house.

The same of course goes for a host of other familiar situations. The thermostat on our central heating system reacts to whatever temperature setting has been chosen; the food we purchase from the supermarket carries 'use by' dates; those same supermarkets tell us that if any item on their shelves is more expensive than at one of their rivals, they will refund the difference. Triage on the battlefield uses thresholds to separate out those who will die or recover whatever happens, and those where medical intervention will make the difference.

We may also illustrate such thresholds by reference to sailing at sea, where the sailor may make use of a variety of such thresholds as 'rules of thumb'. When the skipper goes for a rest in the cabin, he may tell the helmsman to call him if the wind increases above Force 5, or if the depth falls below 15 metres. Any of these can be harbingers of change: they signal possible danger – or opportunity – and the skipper will want to be on deck, should any of them eventuate.[9]

Second, there may be *alignments* or *misalignments* which similarly arouse our attention. This second heuristic involves spatial configurations and patterns that signal access, separation or exclusion on the positional landscape across which we are navigating.[10] Thus, for example, well-aligned buoys and lights are used to provide safe pilotage up winding and treacherous channels, to enable vessels to reach a safe anchorage. The space may be social rather than physical. Entrepreneurs are forever on the look-out for new market openings where they can develop a new niche. Traders look for 'structural holes' across which they can build new bridges, so that they can, with advantage, trade goods, services and ideas (Burt, 2004). The incumbents on the other hand may view those same spatial re-configurations with alarm, a signal that they should bestir themselves, if the spatial barriers that protect them are to be maintained. Examples include John Darwin's account of Asian nationalists, mobilising to preserve an autonomous social, economic and political hinterland, in the face of European incursions from the eighteenth century onwards (Darwin, 2007).

There are plenty of other examples from everyday life. Academics scan funding calls from research councils, looking for any which align with their own particular skills and expertise. The lonely register with dating agencies and look for someone else with whom their personality and interests align. At professional networking events we scan the other participants for those who will fill gaps in our own portfolio of useful contacts, our mixture of strong and weak ties (Granovetter, 1973). We also watch out for misalignments that may signal new opportunities for us: for example, an international alliance whose solidarity is crumbling (Jervis, 1997: ch. 6).

Third, there may be particular *sequences* which we have learned to heed. In dynamically developing systems, sequence matters because it dictates which elements are made available and when, for interaction with other elements. It matters in relation to the triggers and switches that get turned on and off, unlocking potential or closing it down. Particular sequences may signal the proximity of 'tipping points': new – but perhaps fleeting – windows of opportunity to set such novel dynamics in motion: or to resist them (Bak and Paczuski, 1996).

Sequences of sounds at sea serve to signal what manoeuvres a boat is about to perform, in terms of change of direction, having regard to the alignment of other vessels nearby. When we say that something is 'out of sync', we are drawing attention to a discordant sequence that may merit attention. Many folk sayings refer to anomalous sequences in nature (late frosts, rain on St Swithin's day) and the inferences the wise gardener, farmer or fisherman should draw, if they are to avoid disaster (see, for example, Scott (1998: 312) on the farmers of North America). Every midwife and obstetrician (and to some extent every expectant father) checks that the process of giving birth unfolds according to the normal sequence, with the mother being told to wait or push, as this sequence requires.[11]

It is with such sequences that musical composers play and to which their listeners attend: not just in the sense of recognising a familiar tune, but in the sense of noticing how the composer develops a theme, adds others, weaves new harmonies and disharmonies, resolves tensions.[12] The same goes for dramatists, as they weave plots, create disjunctions and bring the play to a climax which resolves the tensions that have developed. Another example is the art of weaving itself: of a tapestry (Greger, 1985), but also of a conversation (Schön, 1987: ch. 2), and indeed of a web of social relationships, with their obligations and entitlements. Those who are well versed in any of these art forms can recognise the key points of such sequences and the variety of new pathways along which the skilled performance in question might next lead.[13]

In short, therefore: thresholds, alignments and sequences (TAS) map boundaries between the areas of our world that are settled and fixed and those that are fluid and contested. The former we handle using the rules of thumb embedded within our habits and settled practices: the heuristics whose biases and limitations are highlighted by behaviourists such as Thaler and Sunstein, but which nevertheless serve us quite well in much of our daily lives. The areas of our world that are fluid and contested need more careful and reflective attention, if we are to attend to the opportunities and threats they embody: and for these we deploy mental models as to how the world is likely to unfold. The role of such mental models in relation to 'slow thinking' thus parallels the role of 'frugal heuristics' in relation to 'fast thinking'.

The boundary between habitual and agile action is, therefore, that between the realms of fast and slow thinking and that between heuristics and mental maps. This boundary is fluid and contested. It is when actors detect anomalous patterns – in terms of particular TAS – that they are alerted to the need for a response which does not rely on the standard templates of the habitual. Just as a sailor uses log, depth sounder and compass in conjunction with each other, TAS provides a set of tools and instruments for navigating this ground and for monitoring its dynamics.

Nevertheless, this is an unhelpful parallel, if it suggests that TAS offers a set of technical instruments and decision-making processes with little social content. On the contrary, it is essential to take account of the social processes by which heuristics and mental maps are constructed, the information in question is mediated and social meanings are negotiated (Breakwell, 2014: especially ch. 9).

6.5 Empirical investigation

How can social scientists study the non-linear dynamics that unfold on social terrains: and which may be variously recognised, misconstrued or overlooked by the social actors themselves? Much of the value of the 'complexity' literature is to alert us to the counter-intuitive outcomes of such dynamics: think again of Schelling's model of racial segregation, or the dramatic reconfiguration of ecosystems that processes of co-evolution can set in motion.

Scheffer and his colleagues argue that there are generic symptoms of complex adaptive systems approaching a 'tipping point' (Scheffer et al., 2009). These include, for example, a slow-down in the recovery rate after small perturbations and increased variance in the pattern of fluctuations. Scheffer's eyes are, however, focused primarily on physical and biological systems. He suggests that financial markets may exhibit some of these same symptoms: and that these can in principle be used by regulators to take early remedial action. Fisher (2011) likewise looks for 'weak signals' of impending change: surface signs of deeper dynamics that are underway. He begins with the natural world – toads and earth tremors, for example – and seeks from there to move into the social world. As with Scheffer, however, his claims are suitably cautious (see also Werners et al., 2013).

Social scientists have watched for signs of anxiety or even panic among the public. Examples might include the reputation of a school falling and parents hastily switching their allegiance elsewhere; a run on the bank or resort to predatory lenders. In developing countries, scholars point to the significance of the seed corn for next year being eaten, or the age of marriage for daughters falling (Chambers, 1989; Bevan and Sseweya, 1995; Indra and Buchugnani, 1997; Carney, 1998; Moser, 1998). These signals are, however, all very much institutionally specific.

Pierson notes that positional struggles tend to bring societies towards critical thresholds. He takes the example of a game of musical chairs, commenting that 'adding a few more players may alter the social dynamics dramatically' (Pierson, 2004: 83). It is when there are just a few valued positions still vacant, that the competition among those poised to occupy them will increase in non-linear fashion. But how do the actors themselves recognise that such a 'tightening' of the situation is developing? What rules of thumb do they use – in terms of TAS – to navigate complex terrains and to tune and steer the non-linear dynamics which unfold there? Which TAS heuristics provide them with an early warning signal, so that they are not taken wholly by surprise? What mental models do they employ to spot opportunities and threats; and how do social contexts and their past life experiences shape the models that they bring into play?

We need empirical evidence as to how social actors become aware of these processes. For example, Goldthorpe and Lockwood's classic studies of the 'Affluent Worker' were concerned with members of the 'sunken middle class': in particular, the mental models of the class structure and of individual advancement that they had formed and how these then informed their efforts to avoid downward mobility, as compared with their siblings (Goldthorpe et al., 1969). So, too, Goldthorpe's subsequent studies of social mobility are concerned with the positional struggles in which families find themselves locked. We need to know more about the critical thresholds they employ, in regards to the tightening of opportunities: by reference perhaps to the latest league tables of school performance, or their own interactions with parents from other social backgrounds at the school gates. We also need to know what arrangements they have put in place to protect and secure the opportunities that they want their offspring to enjoy: and how far these have been made in conjunction with other threatened households (Room, 2011b).

At the opposite end of the hierarchy of inequality, the financial crisis of 2008 has spawned a wealth of studies of how financial actors spotted the opportunities that opened up for them in the years that preceded, but then failed to recognise the warning signals of systemic risk. Blyth (2013: ch. 2), for example, concentrates not on their moral failings and greed, so much as upon the technical instruments and mental models they applied to an increasingly complicated and interconnected financial system. Given that degree of interconnection, what was needed was a quite different set of rules, if the risks taken were to be uncorrelated.

6.6 Policy applications

The world that social actors navigate is one that is socially and politically constructed and contested: not least by public policy-makers at local, national and international levels. By intent or otherwise, those policy-makers shape the solid and predictable ground of our day to day lives. Changes to social and employment policies may strengthen or reduce our job and income security; rules on access to the most desirable schools will set the terms on which parents assess the risks of downward mobility for their offspring; outsourcing of public provision to corporate actors may redistribute uncertainty across different sections of the community.

Policy-makers may also seek to take advantage of disruptions in our settled lives and habits: whether to shift us to environmentally less profligate habits (Verplanken, 2010) or to prey on communities suffering from natural and man-made disasters (Klein, 2007). They may seek to modify the heuristics we use to navigate our world (this is, for example, the thinking behind policies on 'nudge': see also Chapter 8 below). They may also seek to modify the range of mental models that we use: whether by expanding the networks of distributed intelligence on which businesses, for example, draw (see Nelson (1993) on national innovation systems), or by dominating the opportunities for cross-national information exchange (Giddens, 1979: 225–6). Any empirical studies of how individuals, households and organisations probe social terrains must take this into account.

How do policy-makers themselves 'read' such complex terrains in real time; and how do they decide when and how to act? Like other social actors they look out for anomalous patterns that may signal opportunities or threats for the polity in question. For this, they too seem to use the sorts of TAS heuristics discussed earlier to identify situations in which specific actions are needed, whether to reverse or reinforce the dynamic in question. Thus for example:

- The Bank of England is required to target an inflation rate of 2 per cent: any significant departure from this is taken as a signal that the economy is descending into stagnation or is at risk of a self-reinforcing price spiral.

- Workforce planning in the UK National Health Service aims to align future staffing needs with training opportunities: and to offer early identification and additional action when serious misalignments are identified (Health Education England, 2014).
- International bodies such as OECD and Eurostat have an array of indicators of the 'knowledge economy', intended to capture the dynamic take-off of national and regional economies (Room, 2005).

Kingdon (1984) examines how TAS appear to Washington policy-makers. Monitoring of many economic and social indicators is a matter of routine, until one of them hits a threshold that officials recognise as a 'wake-up call' (ch. 5). Nevertheless, as Kingdon stresses, which indicators should be used and what levels are to be taken as critical thresholds are matters of continual and contested debate. Second, policy actors watch out for favourable alignments within the political landscape, between for example the electoral calendar, key appointments to the Cabinet or to Congressional Committees and shifts in the national mood (ch. 7). Such alignments may mean a rare opening for a policy solution that its proponents have patiently kept ready for years. Third, Kingdon describes (ch. 8) how particular sequences and conjunctions of events can open windows of opportunity. Policy actors may seize on new precedents and widen their application; hook policy solutions onto particular problems and current political fashions; build coalitions for reform and undermine coalitions of resistance.

How far can policy research improve the reading and acting capacity of policy-makers? There is a growing literature that celebrates the potential benefits of 'big data', not only to reduce the time lag in reporting on these effects, but also in refining the heuristics and their predictive value. Thus, for example, there are some criminologists and police authorities who anticipate being able to spot likely criminal behaviour even before it happens and to intervene pre-emptively (Mayer-Schonberger and Cukier, 2013: ch. 8). This may not be conducive to just process and civil liberties.

Experimentation is one form of probing by policy-makers (Harford, 2011: chs 1–3). Campbell (1969) was a pioneer of social experimentation under uncertainty: emphasising the importance of trial and error, with a great variety of different approaches. This is an evolutionary approach, in that the local testing of myriad conjectures, with most being rejected, leads to the eventual triumph of a select few. This is quite different from experimentation as randomised controlled trials. That triumph does, however, depend in part on how these different experiments appeal to those in positions of power, whose interests may be directly affected.

Experimentation at the local level may not be able to achieve much within the existing social order. The answer may be to choose a development pathway that also exposes the adverse barriers that need to be unlocked and to facilitate that process (Stoker and John, 2009; Eppel et al., 2011: 197, 201). Eppel and Wolf (Eppel et al. 2011: 186) likewise argue for an iterative experimental-learning process, whereby 'actual policy activities evolve in response to new information from the implementation field'.

120 *Agile actors*

The problem is that different stakeholders involved in implementation may then seek to take the policy activities in a variety of different directions (see for example Hager, 2011). Eppel and Wolf note (Eppel *et al.*, 2011: 206) that 'where the patterns of behaviour undermine the intended direction of change, they need to be disrupted early', but this is something that any of the stakeholders may seek to do, if they see the direction of change as bringing outcomes that go against their own interests. Klein's account (2007) of the neo-conservative project to re-make countries and communities around the world, ruthlessly removing the indigenous barriers to that process, is not presumably what Eppel and Wolf have in mind.[14] Thus the process of probing and implementation, rather than producing convergent agreement, may instead expose fundamental clashes of interests. This requires a judgement as to the value of different possible futures, the interests of the various social groups struggling for positional advantage and the need to call policy-makers to account (Hayward, 2006).

6.7 Conclusion

This chapter has been concerned with how agile social actors 'read' and navigate complex social terrains. It has, more particularly, been concerned with the heuristics and mental models they employ. Just as much, however, it has sought to place these decision-making processes within an understanding of power, interests and institutional dynamics.

Social actors not only probe the foggy landscape on which they find themselves: they may also set out to disrupt the stable ground on which others stand, offloading uncertainty and limiting their access to distributed intelligence. This will keep those others off balance, reducing the leverage they can exert and limiting the options they have in the positional struggle (see also Chapter 9 below). Social actors may also set out to build new coalitions of support and to shape how *they* read that struggle. 'Agility' must, therefore, be understood not only as a skill in dealing with uncertainty and complex system dynamics, but also in dealing with the cunning of an adversary, the resourcefulness of a competitor, the waywardness of an ally and the fickleness of the public.

It also follows that the mental models that agile actors employ are not simply 'technical' assessments of how the world is likely to unfold. They also embody moral claims as to what the world *should* be like; the entitlements and obligations that social actors should respect; and the ways in which power should be distributed and exercised.

Notes

1 Hoggart (1958) provides the classic account of a working-class community in the UK, its settled assumptions and their gradual break-up in face of affluence and consumerism. Verplanken (2010) argues that it is at moments of disruption – for example, when we move house – that our settled habits may – if only briefly – fragment and we may be open to new ways of living. See also Klein (2007) on the deliberate disruption of the familiar by those in positions of power and authority. In such situations of

disruption people try to retain what normality they can, on a changed landscape. To do this, however, it seems that they also need to innovate, if they are to cope and heal (Marris, 1974; Stroebe and Schut, 1999).
2 The most celebrated navigators include the Polynesians (Lewis, 1972).
3 See also Jervis' discussion of decision-theoretic versus game-theoretic approaches (Jervis, 1997: 85). This is also, of course, the stuff of films, plays and novels, where characters are faced with navigating complex social terrains. It is in part as 'case studies' in navigating such complex human relations that such literary products are of interest: also as accounts of how characters and their careers are thereby forged.
4 Chapter 8 below offers a much more extensive discussion of Thaler and Sunstein, in relation to the policies they propose in terms of 'nudge'.
5 For an undemanding and popular commentary on this, see Kay (2010).
6 The fundamental identity is:

$$P(H|E) = \frac{P(E|H) \times P(H)}{P(E)}$$

where H refers to our original conjecture or state of knowledge and E is a piece of subsequent evidence.

The identity then asks: what is the probability $P(H|E)$ that our original hypothesis is right/wrong, given the evidence E that has emerged, bearing in mind: (a) the likelihood $P(E)$ of the evidence E being true, regardless of the particular hypothesis H; and (b) the probability $P(E|H)$ of the evidence E emerging if our hypothesis is indeed true?

This article describes just such a navigation and search process in Bayesian terms: http://cocosci.berkeley.edu/tom/papers/squirrels.pdf
7 Recent exponents of fitness landscapes include Kauffman (1993, 1995) and Gavrilets (2004). The origins of the metaphor are to be found in Fisher (1930) and Wright (1932). This language may be more readily suited to visualisation and computational modelling than to empirical enquiry. Nevertheless, Gerrits (2012) is among those who have sought to demonstrate its empirical utility. Rhodes and Dowling provide a review of how fitness landscapes are being used in public administration research, with Gerrits providing their point of departure, but conclude that its utility has yet to be clarified and demonstrated (Rhodes and Dowling, 2015).
8 Eppel and Wolf have a similar empirical interest. They draw on the pragmatic tradition in experimentation and learning. They are interested in 'the ability to see inconsistencies and be surprised' (Eppel et al., 2011: 196).
9 We may connect each of the three heuristics that we distinguish here to the three dimensions of positional advantage distinguished in the previous chapter. Our first heuristic corresponds to the one-dimensional view of positional advantage. This involved a monotonic ordering of positions, a pecking order, which confers greater or lesser advantage. A threshold is a point within just such a monotonic ordering: of social hierarchies, of ethnic proportions, of temperatures, of dates, of prices, of wind strengths.
10 This second heuristic corresponds to the two-dimensional view of positional advantage. This involved connections being made between hitherto unconnected positions, so as to exercise leverage over the social actors newly connected; or, alternatively, resisting those new connections in order to consolidate and retain existing advantage.
11 This third heuristic corresponds to the three-dimensional view of positional advantage. This involved command and control of the positive feedback processes and dynamic synergies that will shape future pecking orders and connective advantages. Nevertheless, the consequences may be difficult to foresee. The struggle for positional advantage is, therefore, a struggle to offload uncertainty onto others and to build resilience, whatever the future.

122 *Agile actors*

12 There is also the skill of the performer who improvises, for example in jazz. Here being agile means taking music that can be played habitually and finding new ways of spontaneously reconfiguring it 'on the night', so as to create something new – while understanding the musical theory underpinning the harmony to maintain consistency with what is being played. (I am grateful to my colleague Nick Gould for this comment.)
13 Sociologists do not have many tools for visualising the interaction of actors and social institutions. Weaving offers one approach: involving as it does path dependency and contingency but also many alternative new strands to possible development. Weaving also involves ties: ties that are anchored to the fabric already woven, but from which new lines of development can emanate. See also Room (2011a: ch. 11).
14 Her examples are taken from the south Asian tsunami and the flooding of New Orleans to the invasion and remaking of Iraq and Afghanistan: and before that the 'shock therapy' privatisation of public assets, deployed from Chile to Indonesia and from Russia and Poland to East Asia. In all this her focus is on the skill of the Washington institutions in spotting such windows of opportunity: albeit windows that have required a hefty shove if they are to open.

References

Bak, P. and M. Paczuski (1996), 'Mass Extinctions vs Uniformitarianism in Biological Evolution', Department of Physics, Brookhaven National Laboratory
Bevan, P. and A. Sseweya (1995), *Understanding Poverty in Uganda*, Oxford: Centre for the Study of African Economies
Blyth, M. (2013), *Austerity: The History of a Dangerous Idea*, New York: Oxford University Press
Breakwell, G.M. (2014), *The Psychology of Risk*, Cambridge: Cambridge University Press (Second Edition)
Burt, R.S. (2004), 'Structural Holes and Good Ideas', *American Journal of Sociology*, 110(2): 349–99
Campbell, D.T. (1969), 'Reforms as Experiments', *American Psychologist*, 24(4): 409–29
Carney, D., (ed.) (1998), *Sustainable Rural Livelihoods*, London: UK Department for International Development (DFID)
Chambers, R. (1989), 'Vulnerability: How the Poor Cope', *IDS Bulletin*, 20(2): 1–7
Christakis, N. and J. Fowler (2009), *Connected: The Amazing Power of Social Networks and How They Change our Lives*, London: HarperPress
Christensen, C.M. (2003), *The Innovator's Dilemma*, New York: HarperCollins
Darwin, J. (2007), *After Tamerlane: The Rise and Fall of Global Empires, 1400–2000*, Harmondsworth: Penguin
Eppel, E., D. Turner, and A. Wolf (2011), 'Complex Policy Implementation: The Role of Experimentation and Learning', in B. Ryan and D. Gill (eds), *Future State: Directions for Public Management in New Zealand*, Wellington: Victoria University Press: 182–212
Fisher, L. (2011), *Crashes, Crises and Calamities*, New York: Basic Books
Fisher, R.A. (1930), *The Genetical Theory of Natural Selection*, Oxford: Clarendon Press
Gavrilets, S. (2004), *Fitness Landscapes and the Origin of Species*, Princeton, NJ: Princeton University Press
Gerrits, L. (2012), *Punching Clouds: An Introduction to the Complexity of Public Decision-Making*, Litchfield Park: Emergent Publications
Giddens, A. (1979), *Central Problems in Social Theory*, London: Macmillan
Goldthorpe, J.H. (2000), *On Sociology*, Oxford: Oxford University Press

Goldthorpe, J.H., D. Lockwood, F. Bechhofer, and J. Platt (1969), *The Affluent Worker in the Class Structure*, Cambridge: Cambridge University Press

Granovetter, M. (1973), 'The Strength of Weak Ties', *American Journal of Sociology*, 78: 1360–80

Greger, S. (1985), *Village on the Plateau*, Studley: Brewin Books

Hager, N. (2011), *Other People's Wars: New Zealand in Afghanistan, Iraq and the War on Terror*, Nelson, NZ: Craig Potton Publishing

Harford, T. (2011), *Adapt: Why Success Always Starts with Failure*, London: Little, Brown

Hayward, C.R. (2006), 'On Power and Responsibility', *Political Studies Review*, 4(2): 156–63

Health Education England (2014), *Developing People for Health and Healthcare: Workforce Planning Guidance 2014/15*, Leeds: Health Education England

Hoggart, R. (1958), *The Uses of Literacy*, Harmondsworth: Penguin

Indra, D.M. and N. Buchugnani (1997), 'Rural Landlessness, Extended Entitlements and Inter-Household Relations in South Asia', *The Journal of Peasant Studies*, 24(3): 25–64

Jervis, R. (1997), *System Effects: Complexity in Political and Social Life*, Princeton, NJ: Princeton University Press

Kahneman, D. (2011), *Thinking, Fast and Slow*, London: Allen Lane

Kauffman, S.A. (1993), *The Origins of Order: Self-Organisation and Selection in Evolution*, Oxford: Oxford University Press

Kauffman, S.A. (1995), *At Home in the Universe: The Search for Laws of Self-Organisation and Complexity*, Harmondsworth: Penguin

Kauffman, S.A. (2008), *Reinventing the Sacred: A New View of Science, Reason and Religion*, New York: Basic Books

Kay, J. (2010), *Obliquity: Why Our Goals are Best Achieved Indirectly*, London: ProfileBooks

Kingdon, J.W. (1984), *Agendas, Alternatives and Public Policies*, Boston, MA: Little, Brown and Company

Klein, N. (2007), *The Shock Doctrine*, London: Penguin

Lewis, D. (1972), *We, The Navigators: The Ancient Art of Landfinding in the Pacific*, Honolulu: University of Hawaii Press

Marris, P. (1974), *Loss and Change*, London: Routledge and Kegan Paul

Mayer-Schonberger, V. and K. Cukier (2013), *Big Data*, London: John Murray

Moser, C. (1998), 'The Asset Vulnerability Framework: Reassessing Urban Poverty Reduction Strategies', *World Development*, 26(1): 1–19

Nelson, R.R., (ed.) (1993), *National Innovation Systems: A Comparative Analysis*, Oxford: Oxford University Press

Pierson, P. (2004), *Politics in Time*, Princeton, NJ: Princeton University Press

Potts, J. (2000), *The New Evolutionary Microeconomics: Complexity, Competence and Adaptive Behaviour*, Cheltenham: Edward Elgar

Rhodes, M.L. and C. Dowling (2015), *What Insights do Fitness Landscape Models provide for Theory and Practice in Public Administration?* XIX IRSPM Conference. University of Birmingham. 30 March–1 April

Room, G. (2005), *The European Challenge: Innovation, Policy Learning and Social Cohesion in the New Knowledge Economy*, Bristol: The Policy Press

Room, G. (2011a), *Complexity, Institutions and Public Policy: Agile Decision-Making in a Turbulent World*, Cheltenham: Edward Elgar

Room, G. (2011b), 'Social Mobility and Complexity Theory: Towards a Critique of the Sociological Mainstream', *Policy Studies*, 32(2): 109–26

Scheffer, M., J. Bascompte, W.A. Brock, V. Brovkin, S.R. Carpenter, V. Dakos, *et al.* (2009), 'Early Warning Signals for Critical Transitions', *Nature*, 461(3) (September): 53–9
Schön, D.A. (1987), *Educating the Reflective Practitioner,* San Francisco, CA: Jossey-Bass Publishers
Scott, J.C. (1998), *Seeing like a State,* Newhaven, CT: Yale University Press
Simon, H.A. (1969), *The Sciences of the Artificial,* Cambridge, MA: MIT Press
Stewart, M. (2001), *The Coevolving Organization: Poised between Order and Chaos,* Rutland: Decomplexity Associates, www.decomplexity.com/
Stoker, G. and P. John (2009), 'Design Experiments: Engaging Policy Makers in the Search for Evidence about What Works', *Political Studies,* 57: 356–73
Stroebe, M. and H. Schut (1999), 'The Dual Process Model of Coping with Bereavement: Rationale and Description', *Death Studies,* 23: 197–224
Thaler, R.H. and C.R. Sunstein (2009), *Nudge: Improving Decisions about Health, Wealth, and Happiness (Revised edition),* London: Penguin
Verplanken, B. (2010), 'Old Habits and New Routes to Sustainable Behaviour', in L. Whitmarsh, S. O'Neill, and I. Lorenzoni (eds), *Engaging the Public with Climate Change,* London: Earthscan: 17–30
Watts, D. (2003), *Six Degrees: The Science of a Connected Age,* London: Vintage
Weber, M. (1949), *The Methodology of the Social Sciences,* New York: Free Press
Werners, S.E., S. Pfenninger, E.V. Slobbe, Marjolijn Haasnoot, J.H. Kwakke, and R.J. Swart (2013), 'Thresholds, Tipping and Turning Points for Sustainability under Climate Change', *Current Opinion in Environmental Sustainability*, 5(3–4): 334–40
Wright, S. (1932), 'The Roles of Mutation, Inbreeding, Crossbreeding and Selection in Evolution', in D.F. Jones (ed.), *Proceedings of the Sixth International Congress on Genetics,* 1: 356–66

Part III
Public policy

7 Evidence for agile policy-makers[1]

7.1 Introduction

How can public policy-makers make good decisions? What counts as a good decision? And having made and implemented it, how can policy-makers check in retrospect just how good it proved to be?

The most common answer nowadays is that policy decisions, to be good, should be evidence-based. This renders them good in two senses. First, it is only such policies that are likely to be effective. Second, with evidence to back them up, they can expect to command public support.[2]

Evidence-based policy-making (EBPM) became fashionable as part of the 'modernising' agenda with which Labour came into office in 1997. It was portrayed as the contemporary expression of the long-standing ambition, to bring scientific rationality to public affairs. For Labour, EBPM meant challenging established customs and vested interests with the demand for evidence of 'what works': it also meant abandoning ideology.

The Coalition government retained that commitment after 2010, with the launch of a network of 'What Works' evidence centres for social policy.[3] So did the Conservatives after the general election of 2015. The Government's Behavioural Insights Unit has been playing a central role. One of their collaborators has been Ben Goldacre, well known through his *Guardian* columns on 'Bad Science'. He has in particular been a champion of randomised controlled trials (RCTs) in social policy. But the practitioner of good science does well to know and remember the history of his or her subject. Good science also means thinking about the variety of concepts and methods to hand, and which to use in different situations. Which concepts and methods work best in relation to which research questions and problems? This is a form of meta-thinking. In such a spirit, this chapter will suggest three alternative paradigms for assessing 'what works'.

The Cochrane Collaboration exemplifies the quest for sound evidence as far as medical interventions are concerned. The Campbell Collaboration is its imitator, in regards to education, social welfare and criminal justice.[4] This is named after Donald Campbell, the US scholar who played a significant role in the development of the Great Society programmes of the 1960s. That was a self-confident era, with the 'coming of age' of sociology in particular, promising rational analysis and evidence for public programmes. Subsequent decades may have tarnished the promise and shaken the self-confidence. Nevertheless, it was appropriate and telling that when EBPM moved centre-stage at the turn of the twenty-first century, this international collaboration, for the review of evidence in social policy, should be named after one of its most prominent early heroes.

Campbell was an advocate of the careful empirical evaluation of policy interventions. He also endorsed efforts, in some of the Great Society programmes, to extend the logic of laboratory experimentation into the field, using a variety of quasi-experimental designs (Cook and Campbell, 1979). To some degree, therefore, he was a forerunner of the recent fashion for RCTs in social experiments and the careful evaluation of their impact. Nevertheless, even in those early days, the pioneers recognised that this logic of experimentation was problematic, in ways that this chapter will revisit and develop (see for example Marris and Rein, 1967, 1974).

Campbell was concerned with experimentation in a rather different sense also: one that resonates with the work of Popper (Campbell, 1969). In a world of uncertainty, experiment meant the proliferation of conjectures and their selective refutation, as the population in question tried things out and discovered what worked and what did not. This is an evolutionary approach, in the sense that it is the local testing of these myriad conjectures, with most being rejected, that leads to the eventual triumph of a select few across the population as a whole. Nevertheless, Campbell was not naive about the triumph of reason. He recognised that vested interests and the exercise of power also shaped the development of public policy and of the understanding which informs it.

It is with the implications of such an evolutionary framework for the theory and practice of EBPM that this chapter is concerned. It is, however, with EBPM as the assessment of impact that we must begin.

7.2 EBPM as the assessment of impact

The advocates of EBPM have been concerned, first and foremost, with evidence of the outcome or *impact* of a particular intervention. Evidence is collected, evaluated and aggregated – 'systematically reviewed' – across as wide a range of contexts as possible. This is meant to produce a rigorous assessment of 'what works' – and to some degree an understanding of how delivery can be adjusted to a variety of conditions. Those practices with the most substantial and well-attested impact can then be diffused and incorporated into standard operating procedures.

The gold standard of EBPM remains the RCT. It is to this that policy-makers and their public critics regularly appeal (see, for example, HM Treasury, 2011: para. 9.16; Johnson, 2011). A well-defined intervention is administered to a 'treatment' group and the effects are compared with those for a 'control' group. A clear and straightforward example is provided in the Cabinet Office document,

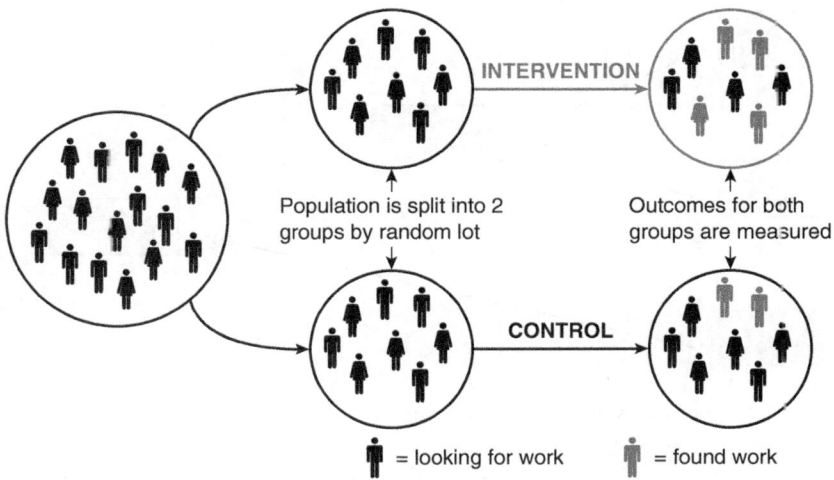

Figure 7.1 The basic design of a Randomised Controlled Trial (RCT)

Test, Learn, Adapt: Developing Public Policy with Randomised Controlled Trials (Haynes *et al.*, 2012), from which Figure 7.1 is taken.[5]

This approach to EBPM is variously elaborated and criticised in the policy literature. Much of the discussion involves relaxing the severe demands of the RCT, successively abandoning one or more of its defining elements and making do with quasi-experimental and descriptive studies (Pawson, 2006: box 3.2). Campbell himself was central to the development of such 'softer' methodologies and the assessment of their utility. Even then, however, some minimum threshold of rigour must be retained, so as to be able to establish 'what works' with sufficient certainty.

In practice, of course, any new policy is launched into a world already crowded with policy initiatives, ancient and modern, whose effects and impacts interact. Nevertheless, if we make some simplifying assumptions, appropriate statistical methods are available with which we can, in principle, partition and disaggregate these effects and isolate the contribution of any particular intervention. Such methods can thus disentangle the combined effects of multiple interventions, against the background of a changing environment. That, at least, is what is commonly maintained (see, for example, Harkness *et al.*, 2009).

We might capture these key elements of EBPM through Figure 7.2. The independent variables X_1, X_2 and X_3 correspond to the interventions that are simultaneously under way and that (in part through their effect on Z) affect the impact variable Y. Each of these can vary (albeit within some bounded range), in ways that our systematic review of the evidence will reveal.

The real world is rarely so simple. Variables exert their effects within different timescales; there may be threshold and ratchet effects; impact may not

130 *Public policy*

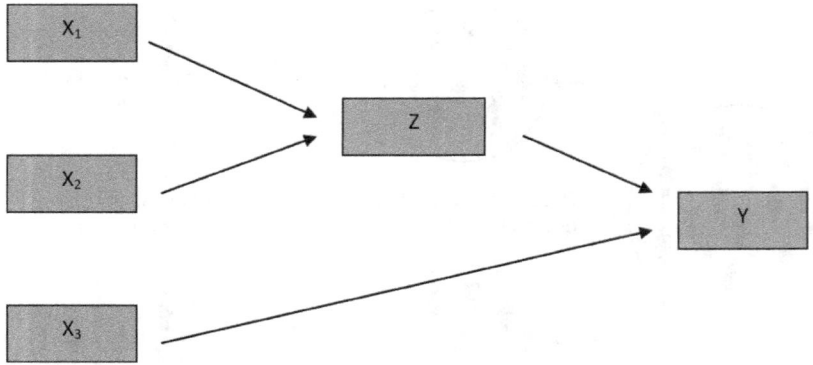

Figure 7.2 Policy intervention as additive impact

increase in strict proportion to the independent variables. Econometric techniques exist for handling some of these complications, so that it is still possible to separate out the effects of these various interventions. Nevertheless, to separate them in this way is more than just a technical matter. It carries an implicit ontology of the social world, as one that can be disaggregated into a set of independent 'variables' that additively compose this world's causal mechanisms. Epistemologically sophisticated methodologies are here being used to trump ontological complexity (see likewise the discussion of the General Linear Model in Chapter 3 above).

Those who develop guidelines for evidence-based policy are often eclectic in their approaches. True, they draw on evidence from RCTs; nevertheless, their systematic reviews aggregate many other forms of evidence also. There is also sensitivity to changes in context and environment. Examples of such eclecticism include Woolcock (2009), Gould (2011) and Sutcliffe and Court (2006). Here are 'reflective practitioners' making sense of their world – and of their own role – through pragmatic and agile reworking of the analytical tools they have inherited (Schön, 1983). The question remains, however: what overarching rationale, other than the RCT, can justify and guide EBPM, in terms which are ontologically and epistemologically convincing? The goal of this chapter is to make alternative rationales explicit and, by so doing, to provide a clearer point of reference for such practitioners.

7.3 The ontological challenge of realism

The gold standard assumes that an intervention can be delivered to a standard population according to a standard design. In any systematic review of the evidence, providing that a sufficiently large number of evaluation studies are included, rigorous measurement of the impact of the intervention in 'typical' situations is then possible. Any minor variations, in the way that the intervention was carried out, are regarded as no more than random 'noise'. The results of the studies under review can then be readily mapped into a pooled data matrix, which can then be analysed to reveal the impacts in question.

Pawson (2006) questions this language of 'impact' as far as social policy interventions are concerned. He insists that such interventions do not so much 'impact' upon social actors as 'engage' with them: both the 'street level bureaucrats' who deliver the interventions and the members of the target population. Such actors learn by doing; if allowed to do so, and given a degree of freedom, they may well improve on the policy-maker's design. But of course, they also have their own agendas: they may contest the goals of the intervention and to some degree bend it to their own ends.

The intervention in question is, therefore, likely to take different forms in the hands of different stakeholders and in different institutional contexts: we can hardly speak of the 'standard' form of the intervention and its effectiveness, without regard to these active subjects. Variations arising from local contingencies are normal, as well as being potentially highly fateful for outcomes, and they cannot therefore be satisfactorily handled by their exclusion from the analysis (Pawson, 2006: 53ff.). Evaluation of the intervention must involve laying out the variety of forms that it takes – and with what effects – under these different contingencies.[6]

This is not all. In the closed and isolated systems depicted in Figure 7.2, all except the measured variables were fixed, and formed the 'context' of the intervention. In the real world, in contrast, interventions not only produce 'impacts', they also re-sculpt the conditions or context into which they were launched and upon whose continuation the expectation of impact was predicated. In other words, social interventions are typically 'open' not closed systems, transforming their world in ways that are time- and path-dependent (Pawson, 2006: 18–19, 33–4): recall our discussion of open systems in Chapter 1 of this book. To examine social policy interventions in terms of their additive impacts, as visualised in Figure 7.2, is therefore at best a first approximation, and one which – depending on the intervention in question – may be artificial and misleading.[7]

On the basis of this critique, Pawson offers a response in terms of 'realism', as developed by philosophers of science such as Harré (1972: ch. 4). Realism insists that it is not enough to establish by appropriate statistical techniques the correlations of independent and dependent variables. Explanation must also include an account of the real-world processes which produce and underpin the patterns we observe. Ontology matters: it cannot be entirely dodged by using epistemologically sophisticated methodologies.[8]

For Harré, these 'generative mechanisms' involve potentialities that are unlocked or closed down by different contextual conditions. Explosives such as gunpowder and dynamite provide the example commonly cited by Harré and his followers, including Pawson. The chemical composition of the explosive provides the capacity to explode, but whether it does so or not depends on such factors as the absence of damp, the presence of oxygen, the ambient

132 *Public policy*

temperature, etc. Causal analysis of generative mechanisms and policy impacts must be alert to such contingencies (see also Chapter 1 above).

Pawson spells out some of methodological implications. Causal analysis is an 'explanatory quest', whose goal is to disentangle and peel away these contingencies. As this investigative journey unfolds, it guides the search for further evidence, rather than pre-judging this by reference to some standardised data matrix (2006: 53–5). Only in this way can we hope for a cumulative and progressive body of theory and knowledge (Pawson, 2006: chs 1–2). It is precisely in these terms that Pawson then lays out a new protocol for systematic reviews and illustrates its application in a series of case studies (chs 4–7).

Figure 7.3 offers a visualisation of this process (albeit the diagram is ours, not Pawson's). An intervention **A** can, depending on the conditions of its implementation, take form **A1** or **A2**; and depending on further contingencies, may then take the form **A11**, **A12**, **A21** or **A22**. The figure tells us that **A12** was the form taken in a given instance but asks us, in a realist spirit, to peel away and reveal the contingencies that came successively into play and the other possibilities that might have been realised.

Nevertheless, this still leaves Pawson focusing primarily on the individual intervention – whether gunpowder or a new pharmaceutical product or a social policy programme – and unpicking the contingent factors that activate or inhibit its impact. We now seek to go beyond this, to the crowded real world of multiple and interacting policy initiatives.

7.4 The case for transformative realism

Figure 7.3 is a tree diagram – a dendrogram – with successively sprouting branches and sub-branches. It is reminiscent of Darwin's 'Tree of Life', as reproduced in Figure 7.4 (Darwin, 1859). In his account of the diversification of species, Darwin

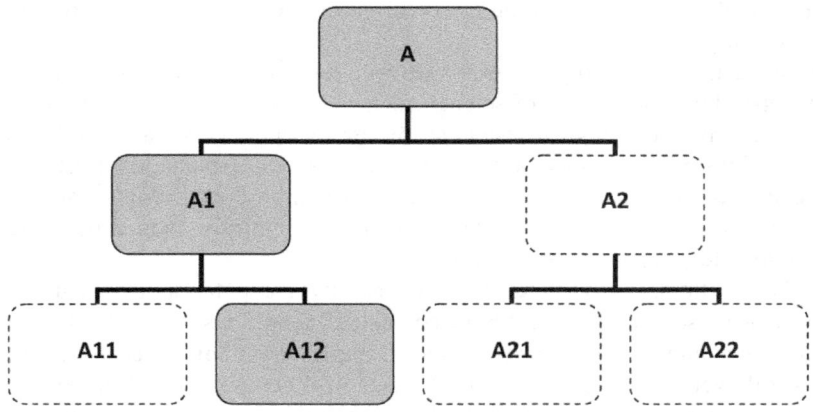

Figure 7.3 Policy intervention as contingent diversification

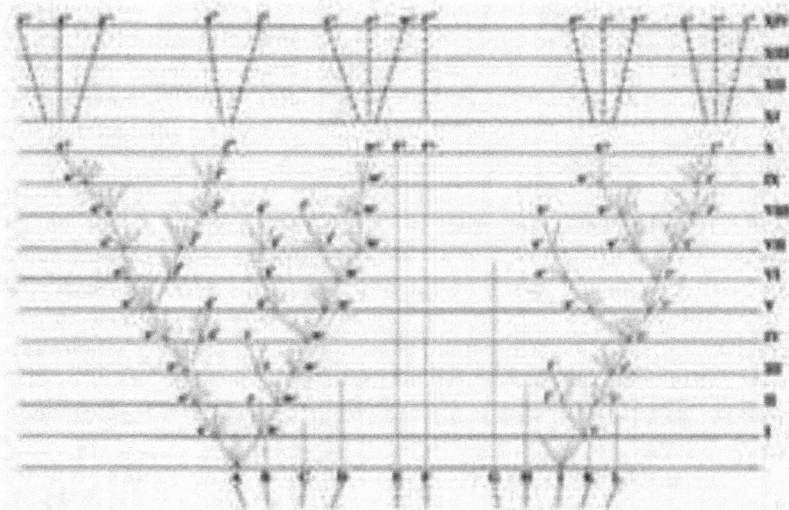

Figure 7.4 Darwin's Tree of Life

was centrally concerned with processes of adaptation to the successive contingencies of different habitats, just as Pawson's realism exposes the successive contingencies which shape a policy intervention and its effects.

Nevertheless, Darwin also referred to the co-evolution of species: albeit not perhaps to the same extent as his successors, who have shown how powerfully the dynamic synergies of co-evolution shape the evolutionary story (Kauffman, 1993; Maynard Smith and Szathmary, 2000). Such co-evolution typically involves populations that are far removed from each other in the evolutionary tree: for example, flowers and insects, mutually favouring each other's 'struggle for existence' over the last 140 million years (see also Chapter 2 above).

It is interactions of this sort, among policy interventions, that we now bring centre-stage. Both of the previous paradigms assumed that we can focus on a single policy intervention in isolation. But in the real world, any intervention unfolds not on a *tabula rasa*, but within a dynamic policy 'ecosystem'. The policy-maker needs to be able to anticipate such dynamic effects – and to judge which ones will accelerate and reinforce his or her policy ambition, and which ones throw it off course. This is critical for any assessment of 'what works'.

Policy interventions are launched into a crowded world. Their forerunners are not the mere detritus of policy enthusiasms long forgotten; in many cases their champions are still at work, seeking to broaden their scope and to occupy the policy landscape onto which any new initiative is launched. Previous interventions shape the fears and hopes and expectations with which the public view the new intervention. Around them constituencies and vested interests will have formed that may favour or oppose the new intervention. More than this, the new intervention is liable to trigger dynamic synergies with some elements of the policy system. These are forms of 'co-evolution' which cannot be understood as the simple consequence or 'impact' of the new intervention. Equally, however, the new intervention may be unable to break into policy ecosystems that are resilient against such new 'invaders'.

It is not just a matter of what policies cohabit a given landscape. Also of potential significance is the order in which they have been introduced. Sequence and timing matter: change them, and the ways in which they shape each other will also change. Not only therefore must the search for evidence regarding a policy intervention consider how it will work in combination with other policies; it must also differentiate according to the order in which those policies are introduced, and having regard to the different time scales of their likely effects.[9] This all requires a *historically oriented* type of 'systematic review'.

This also means that policy interventions and their potentialities are not fixed, in the sense that the chemical composition of gunpowder is fixed. We are interested not in gunpowder per se, but in the weapons technologies of which it is just a component, and whose potentialities, far from fixed, will then be the stuff of desperate arms races. This is an *evolutionary* version of realism. The focus is still on 'generative mechanisms', but these are now located not so much within individual interventions, but rather in the transformative synergies that develop *among* these interventions and their stakeholders and by which they co-evolve.

To use the term 'evolutionary' perhaps holds risks of misunderstanding. Evolution by natural selection is a blind process. In human societies in contrast, people to some degree make their own history. They probe and they experiment, not randomly but by systematic testing and learning (Bronowski, 1981: chs 2–4). They reshape the technologies and institutions of their world, in hope of discovering new dynamic synergies from which they can benefit. They strive to develop thereby their understanding and their capacities; their control over their lives; their positional advantage and leverage. This brings interests and power and politics centre-stage. As argued in Chapter 1, we will therefore speak not of evolutionary but of *transformative realism*.

As we have seen, visual representations can provide powerful images that organise and direct our thinking. Figures 7.2 and 7.3 provided such images for our first two paradigms. We now seek a counterpart for transformative realism, in its simplest or canonical form (see also Chapter 3 above).

In Figure 7.5, **A** and **B** are two policy interventions among many. Each may have been well-specified by the instigators; nevertheless, each involves multiple layers of policy staff and client groups, bringing a diversity of interpretations and interests to bear, as Pawson argues. This process of diversification we represent by the variations **A1** and **A2**, **B1** and **B2**.

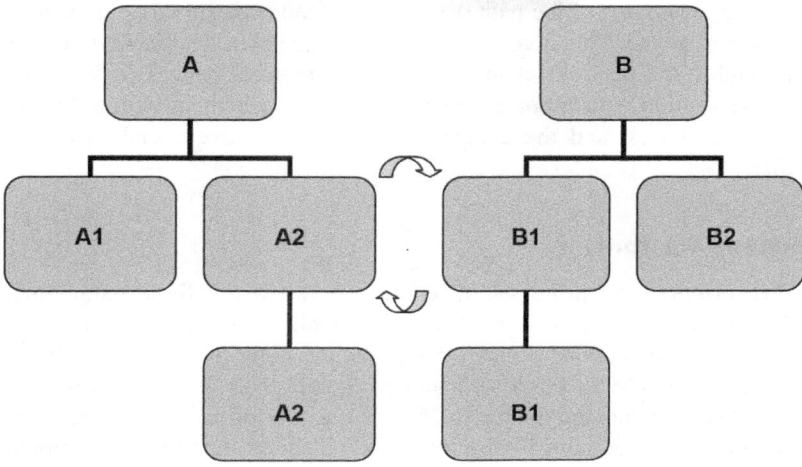

Figure 7.5 Policy intervention as transformative synergy

No intervention is isolated: each interacts with others. What now matters is which of the four sets of interactions between **A1** and **A2** on the one hand, **B1** and **B2** on the other, produces the most powerful transformative synergies. In the diagram, we show the relationship of **A2** with **B1** as being this favoured pairing, this 'elective affinity'. **A2** and **B1** will each now accelerate the flourishing of the other: they progressively dominate **A1** and **B2**, which are reordered, marginalised, frozen or extinguished altogether.

Thus by the time we arrive at the time period represented by the bottom row of the diagram, **A2** and **B1** dominate. This is a policy world substantially different from the one with which we began, centred on **A** and **B**. Nevertheless, domination by **A2** and **B1** will not last forever; further rounds of interaction with the larger policy 'ecosystem' will eventually destabilise them, as new rounds of variation and selection are set in motion. In these new rounds, **A1** and **B2** will no longer be in play, or they will at least have been marginalised: there will be little chance for their potential synergies with new partners to be tested. Sequence matters, because it dictates which elements are made available for subsequent interaction with others.

This is how we may visually represent the third of our paradigms of EBPM, in terms of 'transformative realism'. The task of the policy analyst is to identify the dynamic synergies by which **A** and **B** and their sub-variants interact with each other and thereby come to dominate the changing morphology of the system as a whole.[10] Or, if we take **A** as the policy environment that exists initially, we seek to understand the consequences of a new policy intervention **B** 'invading' the system and re-sculpting that environment; or alternatively, revealing that this environment is sufficiently stable and resilient against such invasion as to remain in its original state.

136 *Public policy*

In light of this, the policy-maker can then set about weaving a new policy landscape, with an awareness of the path dependencies and transformative dynamics that are liable to ensue. This involves navigating a complex landscape: much of what was said in the previous chapter is therefore relevant here. This is not so much an intervention with 'impact': instead it is an engagement with a diverse range of social actors, and the generation of transformative social dynamics among them.

7.5 Choosing a paradigm

Annex 7.1 displays the principal differences between the three paradigms. **Annex 7.2** offers a case study in 'transformative realism', our third paradigm.

The ontological objections we have raised do not, however, mean the wholesale rejection of EBPM as the assessment of impact. Nor do they necessarily mean the entire abandonment of the RCT. It is a matter of practical judgement, how far these procedures can still provide useful guidance in particular empirical situations.

Figure 7.2 will often remain a valuable point of reference. The multiple contingencies of Figure 7.3 and the transformative synergies of Figure 7.5 are not all-pervasive. Some degree of uniformity and stability are preconditions of all policy-making. What must not be overlooked is that they are contingent.

How should the policy analyst choose which paradigm is appropriate? Figure 7.6 provides a suggested procedure. This takes into account that Paradigm 1

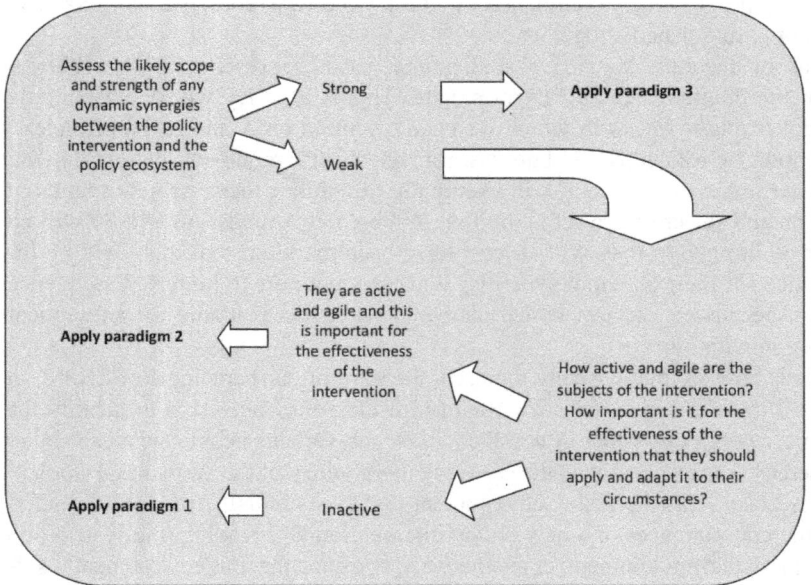

Figure 7.6 Choosing a paradigm

is more straightforward to use than Paradigm 2, and Paradigm 2 than Paradigm 3; and that the more straightforward approach is generally to be preferred, unless the assumptions that underpin it are manifestly implausible.

Figure 7.6 invites us to start by considering whether the dynamic synergies that are liable to develop between a policy intervention and the rest of the policy 'ecosystem' are too strong to ignore: if so, Paradigm 3 has to be our preferred option. If not, we need to choose between Paradigms 1 and 2. As Figure 7.6 suggests, the decisive question now becomes: how significant do we expect the active involvement of the various stakeholders to be for the effectiveness of the intervention?

Finally, however, we note that this choice of a paradigm involves more than just technical questions. It also involves judgements as to the significance of different dynamic synergies, in relation to the objectives not only of policy-makers but also of other stakeholders across the communities affected. The choice involves an assessment of whose voice is to count and the weight each is to receive.

7.6 Conclusion

At the start of this chapter we saluted Campbell, one of the original champions of EBPM and experimental design. As we saw, Campbell viewed experimentation also as a form of evolutionary development. Such an evolutionary framework has inspired our own critical appreciation of Pawson and our ontology of transformative realism. This recognises, however, that in human societies, evolution is not blind: people to some degree make their own history. This is a contested process, an unending struggle for positional advantage. Interests and power and politics therefore move centre-stage, as Campbell himself recognised.

Intrinsic to such struggles is the very definition of different societal 'problems'. Who is to be blamed for these problems and how far is there a responsibility on the public authorities to address them (Butler and Drakeford, 2005)? What standards of evidence are demanded for different problems, as a precondition for the investment of public resources? Which problems require a novel response – and when is such novelty no more than a way to avoid hard political questions?

The struggle is not just for resources and position, but also over the very way that we 'see' the world, both as it is and as it ought to be. It is, therefore, not least, a cultural struggle, over the legitimating symbols that give stability to our social world and the cultural hegemony of powerful groups.

It is on just such a stage that policy analysts attempt to develop an evidence base for policy and practice. What they provide must therefore take full account of the political economy and distribution of power within which struggles over the future of the social and political order are being waged. If they sanitise and cloud this task, in the language of technical measurement and reified system dynamics, this is itself a political choice.

Annex 7.1 Protocols for evidence

	Paradigm 1	Paradigm 2	Paradigm 3
The policy world	Unambiguous problems. A timeless world, where the sequencing of different interventions hardly matters. Each intervention is isolated from others and can be introduced or withdrawn with few wider consequences. No significant lock-in.	A world of contingencies which arise in particular from the active involvement of the various stakeholders. The sequence of these contingencies may well matter: this is not a timeless world. Other policy interventions are at most elements of contingency within the larger context.	Any policy intervention is liable to develop dynamic synergies with those already in place and with others that may subsequently be rolled out. These dynamic synergies are mediated by a variety of social actors. These probe and test what synergistic dynamics a new policy intervention may offer – the opportunities but also the threats – and how these may be steered and reshaped or, indeed, resisted. Scenarios of possible futures must therefore take account of the distribution of power within which such struggles are waged. Any particular dynamic synergy is likely to be viewed positively or negatively by different stakeholders, depending on their interests, goals and values. This also means that the definition of problems is never unambiguous.
What the policy-maker asks	What will be the impact of a particular type of policy intervention, if applied to a given target population?	How will the impact of a particular policy intervention vary, depending on the contingencies to which it is exposed?	How is a particular policy intervention liable to interact with the rest of the policy 'ecosystem'?

What advice the policy analyst can aim to provide	Systematic review of the evidence of such impact, distilled into an evidence base.	Systematic review of the effects of such contingencies, as revealed in previous implementations of the intervention in question	Analyse the dynamic synergies revealed in previous implementations of the intervention in question. Map the local conditions which typically matter, including: • the successive policy interventions by which the local policy landscape has been shaped; • the principal stakeholders who are actively probing the policy landscape; • the social, economic and political connections among them; • the capacities and resources they bring to the fray; • the battle of ideas in which they are involved and the 'mental models' with which they variously operate.
How the policy-maker uses this advice	The policy-maker draws directly on the evidence of the systematic review, rolling out whatever it has shown to work.	The policy-maker applies this wisdom, having regard to the contingencies which he or she faces. Scenarios of the future will be correspondingly varied.	The policy-maker sets about weaving a new policy landscape, with an awareness of the path dependencies and transformative dynamics that are liable to ensue. Nevertheless, it will be difficult to say with confidence what dynamic synergies will develop in any particular case. The policy-maker will therefore have to watch, wait and act as the situation develops. Much of what was said in Chapter 6 – navigating a complex landscape – will be relevant here.

Annex 7.2 A case study in transformative realism

Pawson offers case studies that illustrate his realist ontology. Here we do the same for our own ontology of transformative realism.

Our case study harks back to the Great Society experimental programmes of the 1960s with which Campbell was associated or, more precisely, their UK spin-offs.

In the late 1960s, the Labour Government in the UK faced mounting concern about social and economic conditions in inner-city areas. Policy-makers wanted to know what forms of intervention would ameliorate these conditions. The evidence base was, however, both limited and contested; and the political stakes were high.

The Democratic administration in the US had already set in train an array of locally based action-research projects to tackle inner-city disadvantage. Reviews of that experience inspired the British effort (Marris and Rein, 1967, 1974; Sundquist, 1969).[11] Similar forms of practical experimentation were therefore launched, to provide an evidence base in the UK context, but also to demonstrate a political commitment to address these public concerns.

The **Educational Priority Area** programme (EPA) built on the experience of Head Start (Halsey, 1972, 1974). It targeted schools in four local areas with high rates of social deprivation. Consistent with our Figure 7.2, a novel pre-school language development programme was launched and tested across all of the project areas and compared with control groups. Nevertheless, as Pawson might have anticipated, stakeholders in each project area soon went their own ways, developing a variety of supplementary projects attuned to local professional and community interests. These then became a vehicle for building home–school links. Indeed, in some cases, it was these dynamic and transformative synergies between school and community – rather than the pre-school language development programme or any of the other discrete experiments – that made the biggest difference to those involved: teachers, pupils and families (Midwinter, 1972).

Halsey's review of EPA thus draws together evidence garnered by reference to each of our three ontologies and figures. It illustrates the way that practical policy-making can draw on all three. This does not mean that the distinctions among these three ontologies are of merely theoretical interest. It is, after all, the ontology of Figure 7.2 that is regularly invoked as the preferred model in arguments about practical policy-making. As long as this remains the case, alternative ontologies need to be articulated in no less clear terms. This has been the goal of the present chapter.

The **Community Development Project** (CDP) was the second strand of the UK programme. It involved community-based action-research projects in 12 urban locations. As with EPA, the initial inspiration was consistent with Figure 7.2. However, those involved soon recognised the variety of contextual factors, across the different locations, which affected the implementation and effects of the projects (Marris, 1982). This was more consistent with Figure 7.3. Nevertheless, the analysis which developed within CDP then increasingly focused on the sort of dynamic synergies which Figure 7.5 highlights, in its 'transformative realism'.

The first project was based in Coventry. The government had embraced a theory of inner-city deprivation which blamed high rates of family and community breakdown and poorly functioning local authority services. The Coventry project tested these assumptions, found them empirically ill-founded, and groped for a more adequate account, both as theory and as a guide for intervention. The focus was, increasingly, on the political economy of the city and the larger region and their transformative synergies (Benington et al., 1975).

In regards to the *rise and persistence* of inner-city deprivation, the Coventry CDP developed an analysis in terms of past patterns of economic and industrial development and land-use planning: all driven predominantly by the economic interests of corporations and the better-off communities within the area. This is a picture of resilient inequality, with local and national policies for social and economic development being tilted towards – and co-opted by – those interests. These were the dynamic synergies that had consolidated urban poverty and helped explain why other social policy interventions had not worked. They also helped make sense of the precarious livelihoods adopted by residents of Coventry's inner neighbourhoods, on the margins of the industrial economy and low on the priorities of local authority services.

CDP illustrates how a policy intervention not only 'impacts' on a 'problem', but also to some degree exposes the interlocking array of *previous* interventions. It invades and probes an ancient policy ecosystem and the dynamic synergies around which it was formed, testing and reworking them. This requires a *historically oriented* type of 'systematic review', as argued in Section 7.4 of this chapter.

In regards to *action in the present*, the Coventry CDP developed a programme aimed at re-weaving and thus reorienting these dynamic synergies of resilient inequality. It is not inevitable that policies on industrial development, transport and land use should be geared to reinforcing such inequalities: public policies can be driven in new and more equitable directions. To do this, however, requires the building of a constituency for reform. This is why, in its action strategy, the Coventry CDP progressively shifted its attention, from direct engagement with the everyday livelihoods of the inner-city poor themselves, to political coalitions with other communities and stakeholders, across the city and the wider region. This is intervention not as behaviour change or service reform, but as capacity- and resilience-building for inner-city communities, in their race against time with the powerful.

In building a constituency for reform, the Coventry CDP also articulated *an alternative hope for the city's future*, an alternative socio-political settlement among its stakeholders. It became, moreover, a moral and political entrepreneur, allocating responsibility and credit and blame, and calling the existing order of things into question. This is quite different from the simple model of political consent that underpins Figure 7.1, where it is sufficient, if policy decisions are to command public support, that they are justified by evidence of their impact.

The Coventry CDP may have been the first to be launched, but it was followed by a further eleven. Together they were meant to span a variety of deprived inner-city communities, with diverse histories and prospects. Systematic assessments of their experience – but taking account also of experience in the US in particular – would provide a robust evidence base for tackling inner-city deprivation.

Some such overall assessments were indeed undertaken by a variety of external reviewers (Marris, 1982: ch. 2). In addition, the projects themselves undertook collective reviews of their experience, learning from each other rather than conducting their 'experiments' in relative isolation. The Coventry CDP, as first mover, became the spearhead of that process. The collective story, emerging from CDP as a whole, closely mirrored the account that Coventry had crafted, in its stress on political economy, urban-industrial history and the empowering of working-class communities (CDP Inter-Project Editorial Team, 1977). Only in Liverpool did a somewhat different account emerge: one that gave less weight to the political economy of inner-city deprivation (Topping and Smith, 1977). Here instead was a 'social democratic' vision, which stressed the significant role that local government could play in ameliorating social conditions. Here, therefore, was evidence of a larger variety of dynamic synergies and possible trajectories of development than the one which Coventry had championed. Which of these dynamics were highlighted depended on the many contingencies of urban politics, community traditions and the professional visions held by the action-researchers themselves.

The bringing together of evidence from across CDP would hardly be recognised as a systematic review by present day exponents. It can, however, be viewed as a process of shared learning and experimentation, pooling experience and honing guidelines for practice. Pawson (2006: 32) recognises such sharing as being in many ways benign. It is also consistent with Schön's (1983) account of the reflective practitioner. It locates systematic review and local preview within the practices of a professional epistemic community, rather than within the academy or the laboratory; and it gives due recognition to political economy and value choices. To this extent, CDP serves to some degree as the forerunner – albeit incomplete – of EBPM rooted in the transformative realism which this chapter has championed.

Notes

1 A previous version of this chapter appeared in the journal *Evidence and Policy* (see Room, 2013). I am grateful to the editor and publisher for permission to draw on that article.
2 The alternative to evidence-based policy-making – and the implied target of its critical thrust – is not always clear. It presumably encompasses policies and practices that reflect political loyalties, professional self-aggrandisement or the pressure of lobbyists.
3 www.gov.uk/government/uploads/system/uploads/attachment_data/file/136227/ What_Works_publication.pdf
4 www.cochrane.org/ and www.campbellcollaboration.org/
5 The prominence given to this gold standard can be explained in part by the high status of medical science and the attention given by Cochrane and in the UK by NICE (National Institute for Health and Clinical Excellence) to evidence-based practice. What may also

be relevant is the ascendancy of the 'contract culture' for the commissioning of public services from multiple providers – contracts that need to specify the impacts against which the service providers will be judged, and which depend on a well-established evidence base for such impact (and a policy research community that endorses such an approach) (Farr, 2015). This may also explain why impacts which can be couched in terms of 'behaviour change' are especially attractive, if they seem readily identifiable and measurable (see also Chapter 8 below).

6 When we use the term 'local', we do not mean this necessarily in the geographical or administrative sense, but simply to refer to the particularities and contingencies of a given case, which affect how policy synergies then unfold. This is something powerfully argued by Pawson (2006: 59, para. 3): 'Programmes work in the here and now . . . it makes no sense to . . . aggregate their findings to arrive at a meaningful net effect that applies to all . . . localities'. On the contrary, such aggregation may serve only to cancel out these different effects, making it seem that the intervention is useless. See also Scott (1998: 316–19) on the 'art of the locality'.

7 This ontological critique of EBPM by Pawson has clear parallels with the paradigm of 'complexity', as discussed in Chapter 1 above (Room, 2011). Local variations and fluctuations matter: they may lead such systems into new 'attractor basins', so that they develop in quite different directions. How a social programme works depends on the particular blend of conditions under which it unfolds; to say how it works under 'average' or 'typical' conditions misses the point (Pawson, 2006: 59). For earlier attempts to draw on 'complexity' theory in relation to evidence and policy, see Sanderson (2006), Byrne (2011), Smith and Joyce (2012). It is not, however, sufficient to say that a particular intervention is 'complex', merely in having a number of interrelated components in a 'complicated jumble': what matters are the non-linear dynamics to which such connections can lead.

8 Pawson repeatedly speaks of this as the development of theory and models – our imagining of the generative processes which underlie the patterns we observe. These theories then guide further investigation, in the course of which they are liable themselves to be modified (2006: 100). They also provide mental models of the world, by which decision-makers can navigate the 'tortuous pathways' along which they travel (p. 170).

9 Thus, for example, western advice to Russia in the 1990s, to privatise enterprises even before well-functioning markets and financial institutions had been established, is now widely reckoned to have had damaging consequences for Russian economy and society. Or to take a very different example, popular perceptions of health hazards in light of previous health panics – and the way that policy-makers have handled them – have consequences for subsequent policy interventions, and for the sequencing of communications about such risks (Breakwell, 2001; Barnett and Breakwell, 2003).

10 If the ontology presupposed by Figure 7.2 is of a social world that aggregates additively, that presupposed by Figure 7.5 is of one that combines multiplicatively. Just as compound interest trumps simple, and geometric growth overwhelms arithmetic, the processes captured by Figure 7.5 are liable to dominate any captured by Figure 7.2.

11 In due course they would also inspire similar efforts across the European Community (Dennett et al., 1982; Room, 1986, 1993).

References

Barnett, J. and G. Breakwell (2003), 'The Social Amplification of Risk and the Hazard Sequence: the October 1995 Oral Contraceptive Pill Scare', *Health, Risk and Society*, 5(3): 301–13

Benington, J., N. Bond, and P. Skelton (1975), *Coventry CDP Final Report: Part 1: Coventry and Hillfields: Prosperity and the Persistence of Inequality,* Coventry: Home Office and the City of Coventry

Public policy

Breakwell, G. (2001), 'Mental Models and Social Representations of Hazards: the Significance of Identity Processes', *Journal of Risk Research*, 4(5): 341–51

Bronowski, J. (1981), *The Ascent of Man*, London: Futura

Butler, I. and M. Drakeford (2005), *Scandal, Social Policy and Social Welfare (2nd Edition)*, Bristol: Policy Press

Byrne, D. (2011), *Applying Social Science*, Bristol: Policy Press

Campbell, D.T. (1969), 'Reforms as Experiments', *American Psychologist*, 24(4): 409–29

CDP Inter-Project Editorial Team (1977), *The Costs of Industrial Change*, London: CDP Inter-Project Editorial Team

Cook, T.D. and D.T. Campbell (1979), *Quasi-Experimentation: Design and Analysis Issues for Field Settings*, Chicago, IL: Rand-McNally

Darwin, C. (1859), *The Origin of Species*, London: Wordsworth (reprinted 1998)

Dennett, J., E. James, G. Room, and P. Watson (1982), *Europe Against Poverty: the European Poverty Programme 1975–80*, London: Bedford Square Press

Farr, M. (2015), 'Co-Production and Value Co-Creation in Outcome-Based Contracting in Public Services', *Public Management Review*, 10.1080/14719037.2015.1111661

Gould, N. (2011), 'Guidelines Across the Health and Social Care Divides: the Example of the NICE-SCIE Dementia Guideline', *International Review of Psychiatry*, 23(4): 365–70

HM Treasury (2011), *The Magenta Book: Guidance for Evaluation*, London: HM Treasury

Halsey, A.H., (ed.) (1972), *Educational Priority: Volume 1: EPA Problems and Policies*. London: HMSO

Halsey, A.H. (1974), 'Government against Poverty in School and Community', in D. Wedderburn (ed.), *Poverty, Inequality and Class Structure*, Cambridge: Cambridge University Press: 123–40

Harkness, S., P. Gregg, and S. Smith (2009), 'Welfare Reform and Lone Parents in the UK', *The Economic Journal*, 119(535): 38–65

Harré, R. (1972), *The Philosophies of Science*, Oxford: Oxford University Press

Haynes, L., O. Service, B. Goldacre, and D. Torgerson (2012), *Test, Learn, Adapt: Developing Public Policy with Randomised Controlled Trials*, London: Cabinet Office Behavioural Insights Team

Johnson, P. (2011), 'New policies, like new medicines, should first be put to the test', *Guardian*. Tuesday 27 September

Kauffman, S.A. (1993), *The Origins of Order: Self-Organisation and Selection in Evolution*, Oxford: Oxford University Press

Marris, P. (1982), *Community Planning and Conceptions of Change*, London: Routledge and Kegan Paul

Marris, P. and M. Rein (1967, 1974), *Dilemmas of Social Reform*, Harmondsworth: Penguin

Maynard Smith, J. and E. Szathmary (2000), *The Origins of Life: From the Birth of Life to the Origins of Language*, Oxford: Oxford University Press

Midwinter, E. (1972), *Priority Education*, Harmondsworth: Penguin

Pawson, R. (2006), *Evidence-Based Policy: A Realist Perspective*, London: Sage

Room, G. (1986), *Cross-National Innovation in Social Policy*, London: Macmillan

Room, G. (1993), *Anti-Poverty Action-Research in Europe*, Bristol: SAUS

Room, G. (2011), *Complexity, Institutions and Public Policy: Agile Decision-Making in a Turbulent World*, Cheltenham: Edward Elgar

Room, G. (2013), 'Evidence for Agile Policy Makers: The Contribution of Transformative Realism', *Evidence and Policy*, 9(2): 225–44

Sanderson, I. (2006), 'Complexity, "Practical Rationality" and Evidence-Based Policy Making', *Policy and Politics*, 34(1): 115–32
Schön, D.A. (1983), *The Reflective Practitioner*, New York: Basic Books
Scott, J.C. (1998), *Seeing Like a State*, Newhaven, CT: Yale University Press
Smith, K.E. and K.E. Joyce (2012), 'Capturing Complex Realities', *Evidence and Policy*, 8(1): 57–78
Sundquist, J.L., (ed.) (1969), *On Fighting Poverty: Perspectives from Experience*, New York: Basic Books
Sutcliffe, S. and J. Court (2006), *Toolkit for Progressive Policy Makers in Developing Countries*, London: Overseas Development Institute
Topping, P. and G. Smith (1977), *Government Against Poverty? Liverpool Community Development Project 1970–75*, Oxford: Social Evaluation Unit
Woolcock, M. (2009), *Towards a Plurality of Methods in Project Evaluation*. BWPI Working Paper 73. Brooks World Poverty Institute, University of Manchester

8 Nudge or nuzzle?

Improving decisions about active citizenship[1]

8.1 Introduction

How can and should governments set about achieving their objectives? More particularly, how can they get individuals and organisations across society to change their ways, as a means to some larger public goal?

One method is legislation – for example, on wearing seatbelts or not smoking in public spaces. Another is to use financial incentives and penalties – for example, through the tax system. In recent years, however, 'nudge' has come into fashion, under the inspiration of behavioural economics and, in particular, Thaler and Sunstein's widely cited *Nudge: Improving Decisions about Health, Wealth, and Happiness* (2009: ch. 2).[2]

'Nudge' has had a number of positive effects on policy analysis, debate and practice. It has encouraged policy analysts to move away from models of the 'rational actor' and instead to start from consumers, clients and citizens as they actually are, with their biases and inadequacies, as illuminated by empirical research in the 'behavioural sciences'. It has encouraged policy bodies to ensure that they communicate clearly with their clients and customers, in language they can understand (Halpern, 2015).

Nevertheless, nudge raises larger questions about public policy and the relationship between government and citizen. This chapter takes critical stock of nudge, offers an alternative in terms of 'nuzzle' and lays out the very different standpoint on policy to which this points. In doing so, it also puts in question the disciplinary paradigms which underpin 'nudge' in the scientific literature, and their underplaying of the social and institutional context of individual behaviour.

8.2 Nudge

Thaler and Sunstein start from the difficulty that governments encounter in persuading individual citizens to take simple actions, even where these are self-evidently in their best interest. One example is making adequate provision for their pensions, through the variety of personal pension plans now available. The evidence suggests that individual citizens recognise the risks they are running, of suffering a major drop in their income when they retire: but they hesitate to make the choices and investments that would reduce this risk.

Thaler and Sunstein reckon that in many ways citizens behave irrationally. Their judgements are replete with biases and blunders, they suffer from inertia, they are poor at assessing risks and they are unreasonably loss-averse (2009: ch. 1). Just as a parent nudges a child, they should therefore be 'nudged' in the direction the government deems good for them – and which, indeed, they themselves on reflection generally agree is for the best. Even then, it is not with all citizens that Thaler and Sunstein are equally concerned: their particular focus is on 'the least sophisticated', who they reckon are in greatest need of such guidance (pp. 252–3).

What form should this guidance take? The science underpinning 'nudge' suggests that what matters is the 'choice architecture' that people face (ch. 5). They are prone to make poor decisions when the options presented to them align with (or 'switch on') their biases and fallibilities. The remedy is to reconfigure these choices, so that these very traits will lead them to opt for what the government judges to be in their best interests. The sequencing of decisions is also critical. Here Thaler and Sunstein are imitating the marketing strategies of corporations, who structure the default options that they place before consumers, on the assumption that they will generally choose whichever of these involves the least trouble. The most oft-cited (if somewhat trivial) example is the layout of products in supermarkets and cafeterias.

'Nudge' has been well-described as 'libertarian paternalism'. This might, however, seem a very modest form of paternalism, compared with that which traditional welfare states are often accused of embodying, where the citizen is said to be left with few if any options. Nudge leaves the citizen to make the final choice: government can structure the 'choice architecture'; but if, despite this, citizens still make the wrong choices, that is their responsibility.

But what if the citizen, far from being lazy or short-sighted, is simply but profoundly dissatisfied with *all* of the options which the government offers? In the case of pensions, for example, citizens may have insufficient confidence that *any* pension arrangement will be sufficiently robust long-term, to justify investing a significant portion of their earnings here and now. They may also have insufficient trust in the other institutions involved, including financial intermediaries and employers. Citizens may take the view that government and the community have the duty to provide financially for all older people, at least at a basic level, as part of the social contract with all citizens; and they may therefore deplore the tacit message, that government is seeking to withdraw from any such contract. The citizen may want not a choice, but a guarantee of well-being and security instead.

8.3 Budge

Thaler and Sunstein take many of their practical illustrations from supermarkets and cafeterias. It is from these that they develop their argument that public policy-makers cannot but shape the menu of choices that individual citizens confront: and that they should therefore do so having explicit regard to the public good.

Even so, rather than proceeding so quickly to the public policy-maker, Thaler and Sunstein might have given more extended attention to the role that those supermarkets, corporations and other organisations play, as they nudge and motivate individual employees, consumers and citizens in different directions, which may not all be consistent with the public good. Government may better achieve its objectives by engaging with such institutions and attempting to foresee how their nudges and its own are likely to play out in combination. Thus, for example, Thaler and Sunstein point to high rates of obesity in the US, as an example of the poor choices that consumers make, but fail to highlight the behaviour of the food industry in nudging those choices.

This is central to Oliver's (2013) plea for a shift from 'nudge' to 'budge'. Profit-oriented corporations engage in behaviour that can be socially harmful: he cites the alcohol and food industries, tobacco and motor vehicles, but the list could be greatly expanded. The regulation of those corporations, so that the choices they offer consumers are more consistent with the public good, is what Oliver describes as 'budge'. Leggett (2014: 16) makes a similar point, using the language of 'shove'.[3] But such regulation should surely extend beyond the examples that Oliver takes – such as the more effective labelling of foods – to include restrictions on the lobbying of government by such corporations (something to which Thaler and Sunstein do at least allude; 2009: ch. 17) and the role of media barons in restricting policy debate.

A parallel argument is advanced by Weyman and his colleagues (Weyman *et al.*, 2012). Their research is concerned with UK government efforts to nudge employees to extend their working lives. They provide a systematic review of a wide range of evidence, much of it gathered through the DWP, the government department responsible for national policies on retirement and pensions. The research highlights the role of employers and employment practices in shaping the retirement decisions that individuals make; and the importance therefore of employment contexts, for government efforts to nudge individual behaviour in new directions.

Even so, Weyman and Oliver still tend to view the individual citizen as responding to an array of nudges: albeit these are now seen as embedded in a variety of institutional contexts, shaped not only by the benignly paternalist policy-maker, but also by the perhaps less noble corporation or employer. As with Thaler and Sunstein, the citizen remains the somewhat reactive consumer of the services and products of corporations and governments.

This is not unproblematic. It ignores the active role of citizens, seeking to shape the society within which they live, albeit under circumstances not wholly of their own choosing. If citizens are characterised by inertia and blunders, this may attest not to their cognitive biases, nor even to the choice architectures which confront them, but rather to the social, institutional and political influences and obstacles that they face, in playing such a creative role.[4] This will provide us with an alternative basis for thinking about policy interventions: a critical alternative to the assumptions that underpin 'nudge'. This we will capture in terms of 'nuzzle'.[5]

8.4 Action in face of uncertainty

'Nudge' asks how individual citizens make choices: and why, in particular, they make choices which do not align with their own best interests. Why do they allow their inertia and short-sightedness to overwhelm rational self-interest; and given that they do, is not a benign and responsible government entitled – and indeed obliged – at the very least to nudge them in the right direction?

However, we come to individual decision-making with a different set of questions – and a different vantage point for viewing policy interventions. Individual actors, in a complex and evolving social and economic 'ecosystem', are afflicted not so much by inertia, bias and short-sightedness, but by uncertainty as to how the future will unfold, and what consequences will follow from any train of actions that they pursue.[6] After all, in the financial crisis of 2008 the dealers failed to spot the warning signals of systemic risk (Blyth, 2013: ch. 2): how can ordinary citizens be expected to make 'unbiased' assessments of the risks that they confront? They need some solid ground: a sufficient expanse that is safe and predictable. Too shrunken that ground – too much turbulence and uncertainty – and the actor in question will 'hunker down' and wait for times to get better.

Thus, for example, in the UK both New Labour and the Coalition government of 2010–15 sought to move people off welfare and into work, pressing them to take responsibility for themselves. Millar and Ridge have been following a panel of lone parents, as they move from social benefits into work. The conditions for benefits have tightened and the nudges to find work have increased. However, Millar and Ridge show that the new welfare-to-work regime has only intensified the uncertainty which many lone mothers face. For many, there is no 'slack' for risk-taking in search of larger opportunities: the best they can hope for is just to 'keep the show on the road' (Ridge and Millar, 2011; Millar and Ridge, 2013).

Such uncertainty is not confined to the most disadvantaged groups. It is also, for example, reinforced by the positional races that have developed over recent decades within the UK education system. Both Labour and Conservative governments have expanded the freedom of parents, in principle at least, to send their children to the State school of their choice. Le Grand (2007: ch. 3) argues that this has led to competition among schools, driving up educational standards, to the benefit of everyone. Thaler and Sunstein (2009: ch. 13) likewise welcome such competition.

The counter-argument is that the policy has created insecurity for schools and parents, a race in which particular schools emerge more strongly than previously as middle-class territory. Schools get locked into vicious and virtuous spirals of decline or expansion, with deleterious consequences for equality of educational opportunity (Lauder and Hughes, 1999; Davies, 2000). On such a turbulent terrain, parents are pushed into a stampede after whichever school appears to be best, so as to avoid positional disadvantage for their offspring.

These reforms to State education were intended to expand choice. More than choice, what families may want is some secure ground from which to venture forth: the guarantee of a high quality local school that is available to all and supported by most. However, that choice was not on offer (Room, 2011: ch. 15).

Uncertainty is different from risk, inasmuch as relative probabilities can, in principle, be attached to the latter but not to the former. This is a distinction that Keynes was at pains to stress, building on the work of Knight (Keynes, 1936: ch. 12; Skidelsky, 2009: ch. 4). Thaler and Sunstein (2009: ch. 1) blur the difference. It is important to notice that uncertainty tends, itself, to be socially distributed, with more advantaged groups progressively displacing its burden onto those in a weaker position (Marris, 1996: ch. 7). These include the very people Thaler and Sunstein describe as 'the least sophisticated' and whom they reckon are their prime candidates for nudge.[7]

This goes to the heart of our disagreement with nudge. Shall we view the mistakes and fears of ordinary people, in face of the choices they confront, as evidence of their own cognitive limitations: limitations which policy-makers should seek to understand – drawing upon the best empirical psychology – and take into account, when framing their interventions? Or shall we view these mistakes, fears and inertia as a response – hunkering down – to the uncertain and turbulent world in which people find themselves? In this case the policy implications will be quite different, concerned with extending the safe and solid ground on which citizens find themselves.

This disagreement then extends also to our view of human thinking and action. Thaler and Sunstein (ch. 1) echo Kahneman (2011), in his distinction between 'fast' and 'slow' thinking: what they term the 'Automatic System' and the 'Reflective System' for thinking. The former involves simple rules of thumb ('heuristics'), the latter more considered and systematic assessment of a situation. Slow or Reflective thinking thus approximates to rational action (albeit bounded rationality under conditions of imperfect information). Most of our actions, however – if only because of the hectic multiplicity of situations we face in any one day – have to be addressed by fast thinking, the Automatic System. It is this – and the rules of thumb that it uses – that often produces biases and blunders in our decision-making, even if it does enable us to handle the multiple tasks of the day with an economy of effort.[8]

Here we also distinguish between two sorts of thinking and acting, but set now within a social context, requiring analysis in terms of sociology and political economy rather than behavioural economics and psychology. Again, we start with the sort of social action that is involved in the majority of our actions each day: the 'ordinary' situations that we handle almost unthinkingly, using standard templates and rules of thumb, which we learn as members of society and adapt to our particular contexts. This, Weber (1949) described as 'habitual' action. Such rules of thumb and conventions are carried within the social institutions that surround us: but they vary considerably and are a matter of learned practice, rather than being psychological characteristics of the individuals in question.[9]

When faced with novel and anomalous situations, uncertainty and turbulence, human actors must bring more thoughtful and focused attention to bear. This is what we may term 'agile' – as distinct from 'habitual' – action (see also Chapter 4 above). This goes beyond rational action theory as normally defined. There the social actor is confronted with a menu of options carrying particular costs, benefits and consequences. Agile action, in contrast, rather than taking that menu as given, actively reshapes the institutional and technological landscape on which social interactions play out, so as to reshape the options it offers. Such action involves the use of mental models as to how the world is likely to unfold and how it can be steered (models which, again, must be seen as carried within the social institutions that surround us, rather than being a psychological characteristic of particular individuals). This is even more demanding, when faced with fellow actors who are also seeking to steer it, but in quite different directions.[10]

Nevertheless, for agile action to be possible, habit must suffice for most situations of everyday life. Too much uncertainty and turbulence, and the range of 'ordinary' situations to which rules of thumb can be applied will greatly shrink. There will then be too little solid ground that is safe and predictable: all that can be done is to 'hunker down', wait and hope.

8.5 Nuzzle

In the face of uncertainty, social actors need some safe and solid ground. It is this that bigger actors can provide: whether we speak of the formal organisations – political, commercial, educational – in which we are enmeshed, or the more informal communities – religious, cultural, residential – around which we build our identities. It is by nuzzling close to them that we can keep the uncertainty and turbulence we face within manageable bounds.[11]

From these anchorages we can then venture forth as creative and agile actors, reshaping the world within which we live, if only on a modest scale. Indeed, as well as providing a realm of stability, big actors provide us with new opportunities for enterprise. The birds follow the gardener or farmer, as he or she breaks up the soil and disrupts the cosy shelter afforded to beetles and worms. The social and political small fry similarly nuzzle close to the powerful, not just because they offer protection, but also because, as movers and shakers, they disrupt their larger environment. These disruptions may bring uncertainty for many, but we sense that within this flux, there may be opportunities for us also.[12]

In short, it is by keeping close to the big actors that we can best glimpse the future, limit the uncertainty that we face and devise our own strategies of action. It is also via the big actors – and their connections – that we may be able to access and secure the additional resources that these strategies will require.[13]

Nevertheless, big actors may also stifle creative initiatives, multiply the uncertainties to which smaller actors are exposed and incorporate them into their domains on adverse terms. These possibilities must also figure in any empirically and policy-oriented application of 'nuzzle'.

We will use this perspective principally in relation to citizens, whether acting individually or collectively: for this is the principal ground which nudge has sought to occupy. Nevertheless, this is a generic model of human action, applicable to a wider range of social actors. We can, therefore, anchor our concept of nuzzle within a larger social science literature, before we proceed to apply it to public policies and citizens in particular.

In relation to business entrepreneurs, 'nuzzle' may not offer a particularly novel perspective: it is, for example, well captured in the literature on disruptive technologies and innovations (Christensen, 2003). It serves, however, to underline that many entrepreneurs develop their businesses amid the interstices of well-entrenched big players, not as the isolated Robinson Crusoe of the economics textbook. Nuzzling up to a big actor may involve adopting their rules (for example, the industry-wide standards of Microsoft), while seeking to retain sufficient autonomy to strike off in new directions, when a window of opportunity presents itself (Kelly, 1999). There is an extensive business innovation literature concerned with the interaction between start-up and established firms and the institutional factors which predispose to competitive versus cooperative strategies (see, for example, Gans and Stern, 2003).

Small businesses may nuzzle up to large corporations. However, for most businesses, large and small, the State is an even bigger actor. Keynes highlighted the central role of government in keeping the economy at close to full utilisation of resources and in ensuring a long-term framework of certainty within which businesses can invest with some confidence. Only the State – the big actor *par excellence* – could provide the degree of stability and certainty within which capitalist entrepreneurs and their 'animal spirits' could flourish (Wagener and Drukker, 1986: 38–9). This ran counter to Hayek, for example, who also celebrated the enterprise of capitalists, but wanted the State to limit itself to ensuring 'free' markets and the rule of law.[14]

At another level, smaller countries squeezed between the great powers find it necessary to nuzzle in order to survive, and to find a niche for themselves amid the disruptions those big actors generate. Think, for example, of the years before the First World War, as Europe split into two armed camps, with small countries allying themselves to one or other patron, albeit they were also then capable of causing those patrons pain (Jervis, 1997: ch. 6; Macmillan, 2013). Or think in modern times of small countries squeezed between the established demands of the US and those of a resurgent China.[15]

There is always the risk for smaller actors that they will get too close to the big movers. Entrepreneurs get gobbled up by large corporations; small nations with scarce natural resources risk being incorporated into global imperial systems. Darwin's *After Tamerlane* (2007) can be read as an assessment of precisely those risks, as the European powers became global big movers in the eighteenth to twentieth centuries, and national projects of development in the countries of Asia were variously blocked, subverted or incorporated on adverse terms.

Nevertheless, it is occasionally the small that gobble up the big. In his recent books, Gladwell (2008, 2013) develops a perspective that has close parallels with 'nuzzle' – and therefore equally sharp contrasts with 'nudge'. Now, however, the emphasis is less on the benign protection that big actors afford, more the opportunities to displace or subvert them. Kristensen and Zeitlin (2005) similarly examine, within a major multinational, the motivation of the companies that were taken over. In some cases it was the subsidiaries that initiated the take-over. They did so as a means of developing connections and dynamic synergies on a global terrain, and they then competed to shape the company at large, by reference to their own strategic ambitions.[16]

These big actors are involved in struggles for positional advantage. This is why any discussion of 'nudge' or 'nuzzle' – whether as analytical framework or as policy prescription – must be set within an understanding of political economy: and of the larger socio-political settlement within which they unfold. It is thus that 'nuzzle' points to the economic, political and indeed ideological dimensions of power and inequality: something that 'nudge' largely ignores.

8.6 Policy nuzzles

We now apply these perspectives – and our critique of 'nudge' – to public policies and citizens. For the individual citizen, big actors are initially parents, then schools and local communities, employers and trade unions, banks and corporations and the other organisations in whom we perforce vest our trust – and of course government itself. It is among their interstices that citizens develop their projects for work and family life and for their social and political involvement.

'Nuzzle' shifts the focus from individual psychology to political economy. No less than nudge, it carries implications for public policy. It suggests that government – the biggest of national actors – should invest in the security and creativity of citizens and their social, economic and political communities. It also recognises that the failure of citizens to take up the options that government deems right for them may attest not to their blunders and biases, but to their disenchantment with the behaviour of the government itself; their wish for voice not choice; and their inability to nudge government in a different direction. In short, it turns the spotlight from the behaviour of citizens onto that of governments.

'Nuzzle' also presupposes the active involvement of citizens in the governance of our social, political and economic institutions. It is not enough for government to provide stability and security and to invest in agile and creative citizens: they must also be able to hold government to account. This means government being placed under critical scrutiny by citizens, rather than vice versa. 'Nuzzle', therefore, gives a fundamental role to citizens in policy-making as well as in policy implementation. 'Nudge' in contrast gives them a role merely in implementation: and even then only as consumers, reacting to the choice architectures which

154 *Public policy*

government presents to them. There is little or no attempt to engage citizens as active, critical and responsible partners: they are deemed hardly up to that. That is why Oliver (2013), for example, challenges the paternalism of 'nudge' and seeks a basis for policy interventions that will engage explicitly and openly with citizens.

The popularity of nudge has been evident in the wide range of 'policy nudges' devised and implemented over the last decade, including those associated with the erstwhile Downing Street 'Nudge Unit' (more properly, the Behavioural Insights Team; www.behaviouralinsights.co.uk/). In what practical sense – if at all – might we speak similarly of 'policy nuzzles'?

A 'nudge' is a government initiative that structures the choice architectures that citizens face, such that, given their typical inertia and biases, they are then likely to make choices consistent with what government judges to make for improvements in their well-being. A 'nuzzle', in contrast, might be thought of as a government initiative which:

- gets citizens involved in deciding the choices which should be offered – and within what overall definition of 'well-being' (including the balance to be struck between the welfare of different groups);
- builds their creative capacities and thereby expands the range and content of such choices;
- provides the security and certainty within which they can with confidence embrace and cope with the social changes that will be involved;
- in all this, deals with them not as isolated individuals but as members of overlapping and multi-levelled communities.

Nudge establishes some general principles that should inform any government department, in the initiatives that it rolls out. This includes, for example, that the department should attend in particular to the default choices that it offers (e.g. pension schemes being opt-out rather than opt-in). Nuzzle might similarly require any department that puts forth a new policy initiative to show how the foregoing four principles are being taken into account. We might also expect each department of government, as part of its regular review of its programmes, to demonstrate how far these principles are given explicit attention; and the Cabinet Office to join up those separate departmental reviews. Indeed, alongside the Nudge Unit, why not a government Nuzzle Unit, with precisely this remit?

One example may serve to illustrate the competing attractions of nudge and nuzzle as a policy approach.

In affluent and carbon-profligate countries, governments are addressing sustainability in part as a problem of personal and collective behaviour, exhorting citizens to adopt more responsible lifestyles. 'Green nudges' have become fashionable (Thaler and Sunstein, 2009: ch. 12; Behaviourial Insights Team, 2011; Oullier and Sauneron, 2011). Such behaviours and lifestyles are, however, highly resistant to change, unless accompanied by major initiatives involving strong government action (Verplanken, 2010). Nudge hardly seems sufficient to the environmental crisis.[17]

The race for ever-higher levels of personal consumption is less about meeting our needs, more about the race to keep up with unsustainable lifestyles, as a condition of social inclusion. Attempted emulation of these lifestyles, by the new middle classes of the emerging economies, means that this insecurity is globalised. This only reinforces our resistance to government pleas that we change our behaviour.[18]

What is needed is a sober national debate, as to how our resources can best be harnessed to address environmental sustainability; and a new social contract providing security for all within creative communities (Hoeppner and Whitmarsh, 2011).[19] Within such communities, it may be possible to develop new social practices of collective responsibility for our shared future: building institutions which educate in civic concern and which 'emphasise and strengthen, not the class differences which divide, but the common humanity that unites' us (Tawney, 1931, 1964: 49). Only then may it be politically feasible to move towards equitable and sustainable lifestyles, where we are all content with less.

There is one other corollary. In advocating nuzzle, we have argued the need for citizens to have a stable and settled ground, from which to live their lives, especially in societies undergoing rapid and turbulent change. This does not mean entrenching established patterns of behaviour: for example, the unsustainable lifestyles of the western world, resistant as they are to change. It does mean working out together a stable and sustainable way of living which, in Tawney's words, focuses on our common humanity.

8.7 Conclusion

As recognised at the outset, 'nudge' has encouraged policy bodies to communicate more clearly with their clients and customers, starting from where they are, with their biases and inadequacies. It has spawned a considerable array of changes in practice, many of value. Nevertheless, its intellectual roots in behavioural economics are questionable and its perspective on policy is correspondingly rather limited. We have instead argued for 'nuzzle' as a more appropriate basis for policy. However, nudge and nuzzle also raise larger questions about the relationship between government and citizen. In concluding this chapter, we stand back and consider these larger contrasts between the visions of society they respectively involve.

Thaler and Sunstein (2009) give their book the sub-title *Improving Decisions about Health, Wealth and Happiness*. Central to our critique has been their depiction of the citizen as the rather reactive consumer of the services and products of corporations and governments. This chapter instead has the sub-title 'Improving decisions about active citizenship'. It is true that 'active citizenship' resonates well with the language of both major UK political parties (Perri 6 *et al.*, 2010). It has also been championed by leading social policy scholars (Millar and Klein, 1995).

Nevertheless, much of this chapter has been concerned to lay out more critically the social and political conditions under which active citizenship is feasible for all sections of the community, and the dangers of reducing it to market choice.

The recent direction of UK social policies has been to push as many as possible into the market place and to narrow the bounds of public generosity towards those who remain (Gregg and Harkness, 2013). The very governments who sing the merits of nudge have been passing much of the burden of austerity onto the most disadvantaged, multiplying the uncertainties to which they are exposed (Clark and Heath, 2014). This is the politics not of choice but of fear – and of surrender to the global market.

The post-war social contract, between State and citizen in advanced western democracies, involved, in contrast, a pooling of risks and uncertainties through systems of social security (Titmuss, 1968: ch. 15). The same period saw governments confronting the economic instability of capitalist society. This has sometimes been characterised as a consensual process, the benign fruit of economic progress (Wilensky and Lebeaux, 1958). Nevertheless, as T.H. Marshall, one of the principal commentators on that post-war settlement, warned: 'in the twentieth century, citizenship and the capitalist class system have been at war' (Marshall, 1950: 93). It was only out of that struggle that institutions of shared security emerged.

Nuzzle involves government – the biggest of national actors – investing in the security of citizens, but also in their creativity, and that of their social, economic and political communities. It also presupposes the active involvement of citizens in the governance of our social, political and economic institutions. Consider, therefore, a new social contract with several interrelated elements, going well beyond traditional welfare systems:

- Individual security against risks of income interruption: the heartland of traditional welfare states, albeit in the last half century on the defensive, across much of the industrialised world, in face of neo-liberal hostility to State welfare.
- Investment in everyone's capabilities, not just in those with parental wealth: what many have referred to as the 'social investment state' (Esping-Andersen, 1996: ch. 9). There is good evidence that for a given financial outlay, it is investment in the lowest-skilled that can produce the greatest benefit for national productivity (Coulombe et al., 2004).
- The rebalancing of our economies to provide 'decent jobs' which make use of everyone's capabilities (www.ilo.org/global/about-the-ilo/decent-work-agenda/lang--en/index.htm).
- Investment in vibrant local communities, as *loci* of education, learning and creativity for all: in particular for disadvantaged communities, which are often poorly connected to the community at large (Perri 6, 1996).
- Involvement of all in the governance of social, political and economic institutions, with active citizenship and scrutiny of public policies, and of the 'big actors' whose interests might otherwise detract from such a contract.

Public policy needs to be seen in relation to all of these, as complementary and interdependent elements of development, with significant dynamic synergies (see also Chapter 7 above). It involves a strategy to combat inequality. Just as much, however, it involves reworking the risks and opportunities, the entitlements and obligations that face different social groups: what we might call not the choice architecture but the contingency architecture of their lives (see similarly Atkinson, 2015: Part 2).

Such a contract would involve a broad range of policies of relevance to all citizens, rather than focusing on society's neediest. It would limit the risks of poverty but also promote economic growth; promote individual security but also collective resilience and adaptability.[20] It would rebuild local and national communities, as points where these different policies can be connected up. It would leave the market where it belongs, as the servant of the community not its master (for a similar line of argument, see Hutton (2015: ch. 6) and Dorling (2014)).

This is important in securing public consent to change – by providing everyone with a degree of security for the future, and a sense that 'we are all in this together'. It might even help ensure that the old and mature industrial economies of the west remain vibrant sources of creativity and enterprise, agile in the face of the new Big Actors of the East.

Such a social contract would involve and require re-establishing popular trust in the major institutions – the big actors – around which we variously nuzzle. Loss of that trust has intensified the uncertainty which the ordinary citizen faces. It would both require and develop a national debate, as to how our resources and capacities can be harnessed to provide security for all within a creative community. It would also require a radical attack on inequality. This will be hard fought, most obviously by some of the big actors of the corporate sector: the multinational behemoths, whose investment and location decisions can make or break national economies, and who are therefore treated with such deference and respect by national governments.

To repeat, any discussion of 'nudge' or 'nuzzle' – whether as analytical framework or as policy prescription – must be set within an understanding of political economy, and of the larger socio-political settlement within which they are applied.

This concern with the power inequalities of our urban-industrial societies – and in particular the role of corporate power – was also central to some of the critics of 'nudge' to whom we referred earlier. Oliver (2013) pointed to the alcohol and food industries, tobacco and motor vehicles: and the need for 'budges' that would bring their behaviour more into line with the public good. This critique is also relevant to nuzzle: and to the terms on which citizens are able to find security and opportunity within the formal organisations or informal communities to which they are variously attached. Here, too, government has a responsibility – not least, to 'budge' and 'shove' the big actors in question and to give citizens a voice, in calling them to account.

To promote citizen scrutiny of public policies is not in itself sufficient for establishing some democratic control of this wider terrain. John looks to deliberative democracy ('think'), as a necessary complement to 'nudge' (John et al., 2009) and he addresses this, not by reference to the cognitive limitations of the human mind, but the institutional possibilities offered by our particular form of democratic society. Leggett (2014) places this in an explicitly social democratic setting, informed by a Foucauldian account of power. The arguments they advance align well with what is argued here in the framework of nuzzle.[21]

To achieve this is likely to require active and energetic civil society organisations. However, it is important not to take for granted a homogeneity or coherence of such political interests. The current political and welfare regime 'works' for some. Neo-liberalism is not all about losers; it also produces 'winners', who may not be motivated to support change of the sort advocated here.

The scope for such alternatives is therefore unclear: the main political parties cluster around a narrow agenda of neo-liberal policies with low political risk: and even the turbulence of the 2008 crisis produced little change. Nevertheless, what the 2008 crisis did produce was enormous discontent and a loss of legitimacy for major social and political institutions. It would be foolish to try to predict how new and more radical political initiatives might play out.

Notes

1 A previous version of this chapter appeared in the journal *Policy Studies* (Room, 2016). I am grateful to the editor and publisher for permission to draw on that article.
2 Recent contributions to the debate include John (2009), Oliver (2013) and Leggett (2014), each of whom provides a useful stocktaking on this burgeoning literature. For a useful overview of some of the literature and debates, see also http://economics psychologypolicy.blogspot.co.uk/2012/04/behavioural-policy-readings.html. The House of Lords Science and Technology Committee (2011) reviews the practical effectiveness of nudges but also their limitations, if not used in combination with a range of other interventions.
3 This is sometimes acknowledged in the nudge literature: see for example Halpern (2015: ch. 11), and the discussion of 'behavioural predators'.
4 More generally, Thaler and Sunstein may have moved away from economic orthodoxy's fixation on the rational actor; but they retain its very weak or 'thin' notion of social institutions. There is reference (2009: ch. 3) to 'following the herd' but little to the cues and nudges which are mediated through the social institutions in which we are all involved and into whose rules we are socialised. Instead, the great majority of the examples which they cite involve physical cues associated with the built environment and electronic cues associated with machines and IT systems. In this they remain wedded to a rather abstract form of methodological individualism (Lukes, 1973).
5 'Nudge' has captured the attention of policy-maker and analysts, in part because the word itself has been so well-chosen. It grabs our attention no less than the products displayed to advantage in the supermarket and cafeteria. Thaler and Sunstein – and their publisher – have thought carefully about how we, the educated public, choose the books we read and the ideas which we adopt as fashions. 'Budge' (Oliver, 2013), 'shove' (Leggett, 2014) and 'think' (John et al., 2009) are chosen by their respective champions for the same reasons – they have a rhetorical purpose – and so, of course, does 'nuzzle'. When we juxtapose these ideas, and the competing visions they provide of polity and public, we must not allow the rhetoric to excuse us from turning the ideas in question into a robust analytical framework for evidence-based enquiry.

6 Clark and Heath (2014) draw together evidence that inequality exacerbates society-wide anxiety and that in the UK this has driven the so-called 'social recession', with a decline in volunteering and 'informal kindness'. Chung and Mau (2014) review evidence across different European countries concerning subjective insecurity, in particular in relation to employment and the labour market. See also Orton (2014).
7 The classic discussion of how the social context of different social groups shapes their perception of time, uncertainty and risk is Mannheim (1936), but see also Hoggart (1958).
8 Some other writers, making a similar distinction between these two sorts of thinking within the human cognitive architecture, see such heuristics as an exigency of human evolution (Loasby, 1999: chs 3, 8). Oliver (2013) in his treatment of 'budge' also seeks to draw on a variety of literatures that utilise such arguments. There are, however, significant differences in these accounts, depending on the overall theoretical position they adopt.
9 The investigation of how institutions carry such rules, how they vary, and how individuals learn, practise and adapt them, has long been central to sociological enquiry, from such classical writers as Weber and Durkheim to such contemporary writers as Giddens, Goldthorpe, Bourdieu and Schön (see also Chapter 4 of this book). There remains, however, a considerable gulf of non-communication between the paradigms of enquiry they employ and those of much behavioural psychology and economics.
10 This notion of 'agile action' (Room, 2011) owes much to Crouch's discussion of 'institutional entrepreneurs' (Crouch, 2005: see esp. pp. 67–8), which he likewise offers in critique of rational expectations theory. This we treat as a general category or ideal type of social action. It also resonates with longer-standing debates in sociology: see for example Dawe (1970) on the 'sociology of control'. Also relevant is the substantial literature on experimentation under uncertainty, concerned with the 'mental models' we construct, for envisaging the range of possible out-turns, and as a guide to our choices of action. Notable contributors include Simon (1969), Holland (1995) and North (1990). For an overview of the social psychology literature on mental models and decision-making under conditions of uncertainty, see Breakwell (2014: 104–8).
11 These big mover dynamics are well-illuminated in game theory by a Stackelberg game (heuristically helpful because of its simplicity, limited as it is to a single round). One player goes first and others have then to accommodate themselves as best they can, on the terrain that the first mover has already occupied (Stackelberg, 1952; Tirole, 1988: 8.2). Stackelberg himself applied this to industries with a dominant firm; subsidiary players undertake 'satisficing' behaviour by reference to whatever this big mover has done. As Stackelberg notes, such a market enjoys greater stability than simple oligopoly because there are clear distinctions in terms of size and power.
12 There is a well-developed literature on 'first mover dynamics' (Pierson, 2004). Those who move first into a new market or a new technology may be able to establish a self-reinforcing position of advantage. It can, however, be dangerous to move first. It may be better to move second, once the first movers have revealed the extent of those dangers: albeit what is then left may be only a subsidiary place in the pecking order. Even so, second movers may be able to develop niches of their own (see the literature on the so-called 'minority game', starting from Arthur (1994)). There is never an *entirely* first mover: any terrain onto which we move has been shaped by others. This is why 'big mover dynamics' are often more significant than 'first mover dynamics'.
13 Granovetter (1973) emphasises the importance of the 'weak ties' that we have for the sorts of projects that we can undertake: 'weak ties' being ties to social actors and organisations remote from our everyday lives. Burt (2004) uses network analysis to depict 'brokers' who span gaps across unconnected regions of the network – merchants, idea-brokers and the like (see also Chapter 5 above on positional advantage). It is by spanning the ties and connections between big actors that innovators can

develop their own niche and exploit the larger networks of players to whom these big actors provide access.
14 It is often claimed that the United States, the bastion of orthodox economics, demonstrates the vibrancy of 'free' markets. In reality, Government – and especially the US Department of Defense – has played a major role in the post-war period, in providing a stable expenditure and planning environment for long-term technological innovation and investment (Fligstein, 2001: ch. 10; Mazzucato, 2013).
15 See, for example, the forward planning and scenario building undertaken by Policy Horizons Canada, the policy think-tank of the Ottawa government, for a world in which Canada must deal with both China and the US: www.horizons.gc.ca/eng/content/future-asia. See also Hager's (2011) account of New Zealand's efforts to avoid entrapment within the US War on Terror and the conflicting interests of its military and civilian decision-makers.
16 A final example of nuzzle involves scientific 'revolutions' as described by Kuhn (1970). New scientific paradigms emerge from amid established orthodoxies, developed by innovators who have become increasingly concerned at the anomalies and failings of that orthodoxy. It is, however, precisely their closeness to that orthodoxy that enables them to sense what any new paradigm must be able to offer: they are insiders as much as outsiders.
17 This is sometimes acknowledged in the nudge literature: see, for example, Halpern (2015: ch. 11).
18 Recall Veblen's discussion of 'conspicuous consumption' and the 'leisure class' (Veblen, 1899). We try to 'keep up with the Joneses' for two reasons. Their levels of consumption set the standard for our own, if we are to maintain our self-respect and our membership of their reference group. Those levels of consumption also signal the resources which they have at their disposal and which they could, if necessary, mobilise against us in any positional struggle, imperilling our existence. This is a form of bullying. Rebuilding vibrant local communities from which we draw our self-respect can perhaps in some degree counter this. In contrast, local community bonds are largely ignored by 'nudge'.
19 This is reminiscent of John's championing of 'think' as an alternative to nudge: emphasising as it does the potential value of deliberative democracy in reshaping behaviour (John et al., 2009). What our approach in terms of 'nuzzle' adds, however, is the security and stability which individuals and communities need to be offered, if they are to build more equitable and sustainable lifestyles.
20 Referring to the work of Jane Jacobs, Scott writes that 'complex, diverse, animated environments contribute . . . to producing a resilient, flexible, adept population that has more experience in confronting novel challenges and taking initiative' (Scott, 1998: 349). Here, however, we emphasise the importance of some stable ground and settled habits, if social actors are to be resilient and to develop creative responses to complex and turbulent environments.
21 Here, again, there are useful additional insights in Gladwell's recent writing. While he is primarily interested in individual citizens, he adduces lessons also for the big actors, including in particular the public authorities: the importance for them of nuzzling the mass of individual citizens and maintaining legitimacy in their eyes (Gladwell, 2013: Part 3). Otherwise, instead of aligning their choices with the wisdom of policy-makers (the goal of nudge), citizens are likely to align them in quite other – and socially disruptive – directions.

References

Arthur, W.B. (1994), 'Inductive Reasoning and Bounded Rationality (the El Farol problem)', *American Economic Review*, 84: 406–11

Atkinson, A.B. (2015), *Inequality: What Can be Done?*, Cambridge, MA: Harvard University Press

Behavioural Insights Team (2011), *Behaviour Change and Energy Use*, London: Cabinet Office

Blyth, M. (2013), *Austerity: The History of a Dangerous Idea*, New York: Oxford University Press

Breakwell, G. (2014), *The Social Psychology of Risk (Second Edition)*, Cambridge: Cambridge University Press

Burt, R.S. (2004), 'Structural Holes and Good Ideas', *American Journal of Sociology*, 110(2): 349–99

Christensen. C.M. (2003), *The Innovator's Dilemma*, New York: HarperCollins

Chung, H. and S. Mau (2014), 'Subjective Insecurity and the Role of Institutions', *Journal of European Social Policy*, 24(4): 303–18

Clark, T. and A. Heath (2014), *Hard Times: Inequality, Recession, Aftermath*, New Haven, CT: Yale University Press

Coulombe, S., J.-F. Tremblay, and S. Marchand (2004), *Literacy Scores, Human Capital and Growth across Fourteen OECD Countries*, Ottawa: Statistics Canada

Crouch, C. (2005), *Capitalist Diversity and Change: Recombinant Governance and Institutional Entrepreneurs*, Oxford: Oxford University Press

Darwin, J. (2007), *After Tamerlane: The Rise and Fall of Global Empires, 1400–2000*, Harmondsworth: Penguin

Davies, N. (2000), *The School Report*, London: Vintage

Dawe, A. (1970), 'The Two Sociologies', *British Journal of Sociology*, 21(2): 207–18

Dorling, D. (2014), *Inequality and the 1%*, London: Verso

Esping-Andersen, G., (ed.) (1996), *Welfare States in Transition*, London: Sage

Fligstein, N. (2001), *The Architecture of Markets: An Economic Sociology of Twenty-First Century Capitalist Societies*, Princeton, NJ: Princeton University Press

Gans, J.S. and S. Stern (2003), 'The Product Market and the Market for "Ideas": Commercialization Strategies for Technology Entrepreneurs', *Research Policy*, 32: 333–50

Gladwell, M. (2008), *Outliers: The Story of Success*, London: Penguin

Gladwell, M. (2013), *David and Goliath: Underdogs, Misfits and the Art of Battling Giants*, London: Allen Lane

Granovetter, M. (1973), 'The Strength of Weak Ties', *American Journal of Sociology*, 78: 1360–80

Gregg, P. and S. Harkness (2013), *The 2013 Comprehensive Spending Review and the Implications for Making Work Pay and Family Poverty*, Bath: Institute for Policy Research, University of Bath

Hager, N. (2011), *Other People's Wars: New Zealand in Afghanistan, Iraq and the War on Terror*, Nelson, NZ: Craig Potton Publishing

Halpern, D. (2015), *Inside the Nudge Unit*, London: Penguin Random House

Hoeppner, C. and L. Whitmarsh (2011), 'Public Engagement in Climate Action: Policy and Public Expectations', in L. Whitmarsh, S. O'Neill, and I. Lorenzoni (eds), *Engaging the Public with Climate Change*, London: Earthscan: 47–65

Hoggart, R. (1958), *The Uses of Literacy*, Harmondsworth: Penguin

Holland, J. (1995), *Hidden Order: How Adaptation Builds Complexity*, New York: Basic Books

House of Lords Science and Technology Committee (2011), *Behaviour Change*, London: The Stationery Office

Hutton, W. (2015), *How Good We Can Be*, London: Little, Brown
Jervis, R. (1997), *System Effects: Complexity in Political and Social Life*, Princeton, NJ: Princeton University Press
John, P., G. Smith, and G. Stoker (2009), 'Nudge Nudge, Think Think: Two Strategies for Changing Civic Behaviour', *The Political Quarterly*, 80(3): 361–70
Kahneman, D. (2011), *Thinking, Fast and Slow*, London: Allen Lane
Kelly, K. (1999), *New Rules for the New Economy*, London: Fourth Estate
Keynes, J.M. (1936), *The General Theory of Employment, Interest and Money*, London: Macmillan
Kristensen, P.H. and J. Zeitlin (2005), *Local Players in Global Games: The Strategic Constitution of a Multinational Corporation*, Oxford: Oxford University Press
Kuhn, T.S. (1970), *The Structure of Scientific Revolutions*, Chicago, IL: University of Chicago Press
Lauder, H. and D. Hughes (1999), *Trading in Futures: Why Markets in Education Don't Work*, Buckingham: Open University Press
Le Grand, J. (2007), *The Other Invisible Hand*, Princeton, NJ: Princeton University Press
Leggett, W. (2014), 'The Politics of Behaviour Change: Nudge, Neoliberalism and the State', *Policy and Politics*, 42(1): 3–19
Loasby, B. (1999), *Knowledge, Institutions and Evolution in Economics*, London: Routledge
Lukes, S.M. (1973), *Individualism*, Oxford: Basil Blackwell
Macmillan, M. (2013), *The War that Ended Peace: How Europe Abandoned Peace for the First World War*, London: Profile Books
Mannheim, K. (1936), *Ideology and Utopia*, London: Routledge
Marris, P. (1996), *The Politics of Uncertainty*, London: Routledge
Marshall, T.H. (1950), *Citizenship and Social Class*, Cambridge: Cambridge University Press
Mazzucato, M. (2013), *The Entrepreneurial State*, London: Anthem
Millar, J. and R. Klein (1995), 'Do-It-Yourself Social Policy: Searching for a New Paradigm?' *Social Policy and Administration*, 29(4): 303–16
Millar, J. and T. Ridge (2013), 'Lone Mothers and Paid Work: the "Family-Work Project"', *International Review of Sociology*, 23(3): 564–77
North, D.C. (1990), *Institutions, Institutional Change and Economic Performance*, Cambridge: Cambridge University Press
Oliver, A. (2013), 'From Nudging to Budging: Using Behavioural Economics to Inform Public Sector Policy', *Journal of Social Policy*, 42(4): 685–700
Orton, M. (2014), *Something's Not Right: Insecurity and an Anxious Nation*, London: Compass. www.compassonline.org.uk/wp-content/uploads/2015/01/Compass-Somethings-Not-Right.pdf
Oullier, O. and S. Sauneron (2011), 'Green Nudges: New Incentives for Ecological Behaviour', from http://oullier.free.fr/files/2011_Oullier-Sauneron_CAS_Green-Nudges-Ecological-Behavior.pdf
Perri 6 (1996), *Escaping Poverty*, London: Demos
Perri 6, C. Fletcher-Morgan, and K. Leyland (2010), 'Making People More Responsible: The Blair Governments' Programme for Changing Citizens' Behaviour', *Political Studies*, 58(3): 427–49
Pierson, P. (2004), *Politics in Time*, Princeton, NJ: Princeton University Press
Ridge, T. and J. Millar (2011), 'Following Families: Working Lone-Mother Families and their Children', *Social Policy & Administration*, 45(1): 85–97

Room, G. (2011), *Complexity, Institutions and Public Policy: Agile Decision-Making in a Turbulent World,* Cheltenham: Edward Elgar

Room, G. (2016), 'Nudge or Nuzzle? Improving Decisions about Active Citizenship', *Policy Studies,* 37(2): 113–28

Scott, J.C. (1998), *Seeing like a State,* Newhaven, CT: Yale University Press

Simon, H.A. (1969), *The Sciences of the Artificial,* Cambridge, MA: MIT Press

Skidelsky, R. (2009), *Keynes: The Return of the Master,* London: Allen Lane

Stackelberg, H.v. (1952), *The Theory of the Market Economy (Grundlage der Theoretischen Volkswirtschaftslehre, 1948: translated with an Introduction by Alan T Peacock),* London: William Hodge

Tawney, R.H. (1931, 1964), *Equality,* London: Unwin Books

Thaler, R.H. and C.R. Sunstein (2009), *Nudge: Improving Decisions about Health, Wealth, and Happiness (Revised edition),* London: Penguin

Tirole, J. (1988), *The Theory of Industrial Organization,* Cambridge, MA: The MIT Press

Titmuss, R.M. (1968), *Commitment to Welfare,* London: Unwin

Veblen, T. (1899), *The Theory of the Leisure Class,* New York: Macmillan

Verplanken, B. (2010), 'Old habits and new routes to sustainable behaviour', in L. Whitmarsh, S. O'Neill, and I. Lorenzoni (eds), *Engaging the Public with Climate Change,* London: Earthscan: 17–30

Wagener, H.-J. and J.W. Drukker, (eds) (1986), *The Economic Law of Motion of Modern Society: A Marx-Keynes-Schumpeter Centennial,* Cambridge: Cambridge University Press

Weber, M. (1949), *The Methodology of the Social Sciences,* New York: Free Press

Weyman, A., D. Wainwright, R. O'Hara, P. Jones, and A. Buckingham (2012), *Extending Working Life: Behaviour Change Interventions* (Research Report No 809), London: Department for Work and Pensions

Wilensky, H L. and C.N. Lebeaux (1958), *Industrial Society and Social Welfare,* New York: Free Press

9 Unequal rewards and the super-rich

9.1 Introduction

How shall we make sense of the high and growing levels of inequality that have become apparent during recent decades within the countries of the western world, notably the US and the UK (Congressional Budget Office, 2013: ch. 10)? One aspect is the growing disparity between the share of labour and capital in national income. In almost all OECD nations, over the last three decades, the share going to capital has increased greatly. Another is growing income inequality within the population, reflecting in part the higher rewards going to capital owners and business elites and the higher wages of the better educated.[1] Alongside this growing inequality in income, disparities of wealth have also been widening (Hills *et al.*, 2013; Dorling, 2014: ch. 4; Atkinson, 2015: ch. 1; Sayer, 2015).

Piketty's highly influential *Capital in the Twenty-First Century* (2014) warns that capitalism has an in-built tendency to such growing inequality. We cannot rely on wealth and prosperity to 'trickle down'. Nor can we take comfort from the 'Kuznets curve', predicting that while inequality is likely to be high in the early stages of development, it will then progressively fall. It is true that inequalities of capital ownership and income from capital fell in the period 1914–45; but this he argues was due to the destruction of wealth in two world wars and the social and political turmoil of the time. Now, however, old trends in inequality have re-asserted themselves. What is needed, Piketty argues, is purposeful government action to reduce such inequalities: without these, the future of our societies is unlikely to be pleasant. However, Piketty's own analysis is not without flaw (Room, 2015a).

Sociologists and political scientists have also sought to make sense of this winner-takes-all society (Hacker and Pierson, 2010; Crouch, 2011). In explaining the high levels of reward that have been captured by corporate elites in recent decades, they point to their opportunistic looting and predation. This is echoed by various renegade economists (Galbraith, 2009; Smith, 2010). Even so, it remains to be explained how it was that these particular individuals – rather than anyone else – got to be in such enviable positions; how these extravagant rewards came to be seen as reasonable and legitimate to the actors involved; and to what degree such a winner-takes-all society is a matter of public policy choices.

This chapter considers what light may be shed by the account of complex and contingent dynamics offered in the previous chapters, set within an understanding of political economy: and the implications for public policy and social justice. However, the rich include groups with diverse forms and combinations of income and wealth, albeit united in defence and celebration of their shared position and accomplishments (Piketty, 2014: 301). This makes it more complicated to decide what we are talking about and to disentangle the various elements. This tangle also makes it easier for elements of the super-rich with more dubious justifications for their assets to borrow respectability from those whose claims seem more robust and heroic. It is these interconnections that we shall endeavour to illuminate.

We start however with conventional explanations of unequal rewards.

9.2 Inequality on stable and settled ground

Within mainstream economics, the most widely embraced explanation of differential rewards is in terms of a worker's marginal product. The wage received equates to the net value of the extra output resulting from the worker's efforts.[2] This explanation seems clear: it also seems to provide a normative justification for inequalities of reward with which few could disagree. Nevertheless, this simple equation involves a number of assumptions.

It assumes, first, that labour markets are efficient and will allow employers to attract additional workers, by raising the wage they are prepared to pay. It assumes, second, that the extra output that each additional worker produces will steadily fall, if the capital stock of the enterprise remains unchanged. With wages edging upwards and the value of the additional output per worker edging down, the enterprise will expand its labour force until the wage matches the value of that marginal product.

Admittedly it may be hard to determine what that marginal product is (other than by inferring it from the payment received); but we can rest assured that the market will enforce this equivalence, whether or not we are able to check this empirically. Or, at the very least, we are entitled to conclude that this equivalence will tend increasingly to apply, the more we liberate markets from frictions, imperfect information and monopoly elements (all factors which mainstream economists have sought to address). Among the latter are the restrictions imposed by professions and trade unions: hence the opprobrium such groups tend to attract from the champions of 'free' markets.

Each person, therefore, earns the return on their skills and their productive contribution that efficient markets and the existing technology impose – no more and no less – except insofar as self-interested cartels develop, constraining the free operation of the market. It is from this starting point that various further strands of the social and economic literature have then built. There is, first, a literature on skills and human capital. This portrays rational individuals as investing time in education and training, so as to acquire scarce skills, with a view to entering the labour market and employment at a correspondingly higher skill level.

Their marginal products will now be greater, as therefore will their financial remuneration also (Becker, 1964; Mincer, 1974).

In the 1960s, sociological theories in the functionalist tradition, especially in the United States, generalised this account, to depict an individualistic, competitive and meritocratic society, which combined economic efficiency with social equity (Blau and Duncan, 1967; Bell, 1974). More recently, there has been concern that economic growth and technological change may be 'skill-biased', with only those with high levels of ability and skills able to maintain secure and well-rewarded employment, while the rest are left to eke out a more precarious existence (Brown et al., 2011).

This explanation of differential rewards is supposed to apply to the corporate elite as much as it does to ordinary workers. It is nevertheless difficult to assess the marginal product of managers, given that they are a line item, an overhead, a fixed cost (Piketty, 2014: 330ff.). An alternative theory takes managers to be paid by reference to the amount of activity for which they are responsible: as indicated, for example, by the number of people below them in the hierarchy – or the size of the balance sheet. This is less a market process than a bureaucratic process. Nevertheless, it maintains the assumption that the individuals in question are being paid by reference to their efforts and skills: with efficient and competitive labour markets – or procedures and conventions that will produce equivalent outcomes – ensuring that the most skilled candidates are channelled into the positions in question.

Mainstream economics supposes that what applies to individuals applies equally to capital itself: and that this also earns a reward corresponding to its marginal product. The income stream passing to the owners of capital is thus to be understood as analogous to that passing to the worker: and to be similarly shaped by the impersonal logic of markets and technology.[3] Nevertheless, as in the case of labour, self-interested cartels may interfere with the impersonal determination of rewards by the market. Hence the efforts by public regulators to promote competition, lest monopoly power attracts excess profit.

In all the foregoing, the differentiation of rewards is assumed to develop across a rather stable and settled terrain. The capital stock of the enterprise is taken as given: markets and selection processes are well-grounded. Notice, however, that an explanation that may seem robust in relation to individual workers is extended to explain the rewards earned by managers and by capital itself, notwithstanding the heroic theoretical assumptions that this entails. Notice also how the *explanation* of differential rewards can easily morph into a normative *justification* for the particular differentials that empirically prevail.[4]

9.3 Inequality under conditions of dynamic and disruptive change

Explanations of rewards in terms of marginal products assume given technologies, well-functioning markets and generally stable conditions: albeit their proponents then extend them to economies enjoying stable growth and technical progress

(Hahn and Matthews, 1965). There is a separate strand of economic theorising concerned with rewards under conditions of dynamic and disruptive change. It points us to the risks and rewards of entrepreneurship, as innovators develop the technologies of the future, with some achieving market success, even if many others fail.

Here we find Keynes (1936) and his account of the 'animal spirits' of capitalists; Schumpeter and 'creative destruction'; Marx and capitalist accumulation (Wagener and Drukker, 1986). Here is the literature on innovation and the conditions under which innovation can 'take off' and produce a fundamental shift in our technologies, markets and products (Rogers, 2003). Here also is the literature on technological innovation within the economy seen as an evolving system (Potts, 2000; Beinhocker, 2007). Technological innovations are continuously generated by myriad entrepreneurs, no less than the 'variations' highlighted by Darwin as the dynamic of evolutionary change in nature. Here, however, it is markets that provide the blind selective environment that decides which of these innovations is taken up by the wider population, leaving others to wither.

The risks of failure are high. Entrepreneurs produce a proliferation of novelties but they must be prepared to see most of them tried and rejected by the population at large. The rationality of the entrepreneur on this foggy landscape is severely bounded: nobody has a rational basis for 'picking winners'. The few who do succeed can well claim that whatever gains they make are an appropriate and just compensation for having taken those risks.

Writers such as Potts and Beinhocker have much in common with our own use of evolutionary perspectives: their work appeared in Chapter 2 above. Nevertheless, we argued that in the social world the process of selection is by no means as 'blind' as in the natural world. Entrepreneurs may be able to shape the market: power and vested interests matter. They may also seek to perpetuate their intellectual property rights in the innovation. This, as Sayer (2015: Part 1) argues, may be better described as wealth extraction rather than wealth creation.

Enterprise and risk-taking are not matters for the innovators alone. The costs of disruptive change may fall on a wide range of other social groups, including those who are least able to bear them: capitalist societies typically leave such groups to be protected, if at all, by the public purse (Hirschman, 1958). It is also important to recognise that enterprise and innovation benefit from the social and institutional contexts within which they develop and from many public policies, including on education, research and development, transport infrastructures, legal and commercial systems, etc. Here we find Lundvall *et al.* (2006) on 'national innovation systems' and Mazzucato (2013) on the 'entrepreneurial state'. The latter questions whether risk-taking entrepreneurs should be free to take whatever winnings they can: arguing instead that enterprise and innovation presuppose a well-ordered society and a variety of public goods and that for these, the community is entitled to reap a dividend.

The literature we reviewed in the previous section assumed 'diminishing returns': that is to say, with a given capital stock, the extra output that each additional worker produces will steadily fall. This assumption is commonly adopted in orthodox economics, as a condition for modelling the stability of markets. There is, however, another important strand of the economics literature that accepts 'increasing returns' as a common feature of a market economy (Toner, 1999). These can produce self-reinforcing processes of change, which generate huge rewards, but also disrupt existing technologies and productive activities. This is captured by the literature on 'first movers' and 'winner-takes all dynamics' (Frank and Cook, 1995).

Thus Brynjolfsson and McAfee (2014: chs 9–11) celebrate the way that digitisation and IT systems can vastly increase the economic surplus available to companies that win out, reducing the workforce required and forcing professions and companies to transform or die. Some of this surplus represents the reward for technological innovation; some the enhanced and almost costless throughput of services that scaling-up permits. Windfalls may also arise from dynamic and disruptive changes to market structures and regulatory systems. Over recent decades these have included waves of corporate mergers and consolidations, the privatisation of public services and the waves of new financial 'products' that came to popular attention in the aftermath of the 2008 financial crisis and bailouts (Sayer 2015: chs 4, 7).

9.4 Rewards and their justification

We have reviewed two explanations of unequal rewards. One assumes generally stable conditions in terms of technologies and markets: it explains in terms of their marginal products the rewards received by workers with different levels of skill. The other is concerned with conditions of dynamic and disruptive change: it explains the rewards of entrepreneurs and innovators by reference to their risk-taking.

As analytic approaches, both of these make rather a lot of assumptions, as to how the empirical world actually works. Even so, their proponents have been enthusiastic in extending their application significantly beyond their original domains. Not least, they have been variously applied to the question with which we started: how to make sense of the enormous rewards that have accrued to the very wealthy in recent decades?

The explanation and the justification of reward differentials rarely part company. Each of the foregoing explanations has been taken as also justifying the prevailing inequalities: at least in the sense of suggesting that no alternative would be workable. There is little basis for protesting at any of these inequalities, if they are the inevitable result of necessary processes. It can however be argued against this, that the rewards accruing to different groups are matters of negotiation and argument, even if they take those 'hard' factors as a key point of reference. Rewards are a matter for interrogation and critical discussion, aimed at exposing their rationale (see Chapter 4 above): weighing the significance of those 'hard' factors, but also advancing a range of moral claims and evoking various notions of social justice, entitlement and obligation.

This was a central argument of Wootton's (1955) *Social Foundations of Wages Policy* in the immediate post-war period. More recently, it has been argued by Avent-Holt and Tomaskovic-Devey (2013). Different groups of employees band together and weave broad categorical distinctions which support their status claims, by reference to their allegedly unique features. The human capital with which workers are endowed is now best seen, not as measuring their contribution to productivity, but as providing internal bargaining chips and status claims. The external environment provides a further point of reference for such claims: including for example the rewards won by similar groups of workers elsewhere, and the tightness of the market for their skills (DiPrete et al., 2010).

Across much of the economy, these negotiations over rewards stabilise into routines and practices that may not be regarded by all as entirely justified, but which are nevertheless accepted, albeit grudgingly, given the balance of power across the industry in question and within society as a whole. It is, however, when new areas of activity develop, disrupting those stable conditions, that these routines are liable to break down or be actively contested. The various groups of actors involved are then likely to struggle for advantage on this newly contested terrain: whether to seize new opportunities for advance, or to limit the extent to which their established position is undermined. This struggle is likely to be concerned as much with the new routines and practices to be adopted within these new arenas, as with the distribution of rewards as such.

Goldthorpe, in a paper written in the 1960s, considered the anomic state of British industrial relations (Goldthorpe, 1974). A period of low unemployment had shifted the balance of power towards organised labour; groups of workers pressed home their advantage, in terms of their wage demands, in disregard of national collective bargaining agreements. In these changed conditions, no stable normative systems appropriate to this new balance of power had emerged: disorder prevailed. Goldthorpe went on to argue that to restore order in the wage-bargaining process would be no simple matter, given the gross inequalities prevailing in British society at large and their lack of normative justification.

In retrospect, his argument takes on additional significance in light of the failure of the Labour Government of 1974–9 to establish such order and the subsequent triumph of the Thatcher revolution. That led to a very different world, of high unemployment and weakened trade unions. Now it was corporate interests and the more advantaged sections of society that were able to defend their positions of advantage: and not only to defend, but also to extend them, across a variety of socio-economic terrains, from education to the labour market, to the social security system and the housing market (Goldthorpe, 1978, 1984, 1985). This was normative struggle driven from a quite different direction.

Fligstein (2001) is similarly concerned with corporate interests and how, in particular, US corporations handled disruptions and transitions during the last third of the twentieth century. The challenge was to establish and maintain stable patterns of social organisation, both internally and externally, and to address the *anomie* that emerged in novel conditions. The task was thus a cultural project, but one that involved a fundamental struggle for dominance. Fligstein examines, for example, the organisational cultures of financial control that became prevalent in US business in the 1980s. These then provided the vantage point from which corporate actors grappled with new arenas as they became available, including the newly privatised public services.

We referred earlier to the windfalls that may arise from the disruption to established arenas. The very speed of these changes tends to mean that new and stable norms have little time to develop in relation to the distribution of such surpluses. It may, therefore, be not so much the *size* of such windfalls that explains the enormous rewards accruing to those already rich, but rather the anomic environment for claim-making that such turbulence typically produces. Entrepreneurs may best be able to extract advantage, not so much through continuing technological innovation, as by perpetuating such a situation of *anomie*. With few navigational aids for judging what claims are reasonable, it is hardly surprising if – before other claimants have an opportunity to argue their own desserts – those in command leap to pay themselves generously, and to construct justifications for such generosity, using whatever normative *bricolage* lies conveniently to hand (Sayer, 2015: chs 2, 13). This is a rather clear exercise of their power, not least in imposing this normative – and indeed ideological – legitimation of their desserts (Lukes, 2005). Other social actors may have little option but to hunker down and accept such a *fait accompli*.

9.5 Building positional advantage

We have so far been concerned with two orthodox explanations of unequal rewards. Each of them makes reference to technology: whether the marginal product of a stable technology and production function, or the entrepreneurial risks of technological innovation. We have pointed, however, to the role of normative rationales as against technological imperatives; more generally we have questioned the relevance of either of these explanations as applied to elite rewards in today's world.

An alternative vantage point is needed. We now seek an explanation of unequal rewards, which builds on our account in previous chapters of agile action and an appreciation of the larger processes of structural change that are under way at a macro-level – and within which windfalls can be discovered. This will be an account of contingent historical change of the sort with which Chapter 3 was concerned. It will consider how social actors probe novel situations, but drawing on practices and mental models honed on familiar and settled ground: recall our discussion of agile action in Chapter 4. It will build on the discussion, in Chapter 5, of the various positions of advantage and disadvantage in which social actors find themselves – and from which they lever new opportunities, or divert emerging threats onto others. It will consider – as we did in Chapter 6 – how social actors navigate these complex and foggy terrains and how they shape the allocation of rewards within these novel arenas. It will resonate with our account in Chapter 1 of the emergence of organised regularities from social micro-interactions – but always set within an institutional setting and political economy through which power is exercised.

Agile opportunism and 'luck'

In his book, *Outliers*, Gladwell (2008) notices how the selection processes that our societies use to identify candidates for educational and training opportunities often include elements that are unintentionally arbitrary. True, those opportunities may then produce a cohort of outstanding performers: but had others been selected, this would probably have been just as true.

In Canadian schools, hockey coaches each year make an assessment as to which youngsters are showing most aptitude for the sport and should be offered elite training opportunities. This selection does not take account of when the child's birthday falls. However, those who are youngest in the age cohort tend of course to be smaller and less strong: they are therefore less likely to be selected. The door to elite hockey training is thereafter closed to them. Those who are selected then have a great deal of time and support invested in them; the high level of performance they attain seems to validate the whole process. Nevertheless, the selection process inadvertently neglects many who have no less talent that might similarly have been nurtured. This is not a good use of human potential.[5]

Gladwell argues that the most 'successful' of people are typically those who happen to have benefitted from a succession of such contingent selection processes. Most obviously, much of our educational system is organised in terms of the Matthew principle: at each stage, it is those who succeed who are then offered further opportunities. This makes for highly unequal investments, as far as different children's educational experience as a whole is concerned.

Of course, the individuals in question – the 'high fliers' – will typically have been agile opportunists as well, working long hours and discovering smart shortcuts. They will therefore readily feel that their success has been the result of their own efforts, in fair competition with their peers. Most of them will also have been helped by the agility of their parents, using their money and their social networks to seize ladders that might otherwise have passed unnoticed, and to rescue their offspring from snakes down which they might otherwise have fallen (for example, when the local police caught them taking drugs or speeding).

Meanwhile, however, there is robust and longstanding evidence that the 'low fliers' come disproportionately from homes and communities which tend to reinforce their disadvantage (Halsey, 1972). This helps explain why the relative mobility chances of those born into different social classes remain highly unequal, with family financial and social capital continuing to count for a lot (Goldthorpe and Mills, 2008). This all tends to produce a 'winner-takes-all' society, with divisions of inclusion and exclusion that deepen over the life-course: a race involving cumulative contingency, but run on increasingly unequal terms. Nevertheless, there is always some scope for public policies to churn up the competition or to moderate the gradient of such inequality.

Closed doors and unexpected openings

Closed doors sometimes bring other types of opportunity. The youngsters selected for elite hockey training will thereafter have little time for other pursuits. Those who miss out however, because of their birth dates, now have time on their hands for other opportunities that may come along. These may take them along the pathway to becoming an international pianist, an IT whizz-kid or a gangland godfather. Success at hockey is not the only measure of fulfilment, or the only pathway to high financial reward.

During the first half of the twentieth century, Jewish law firms in New York were excluded from the business opportunities dominated by the largest and most successful law firms, led by the Anglo-Saxon elite (Gladwell, 2008: 116–28). They therefore had to work on marginal issues, such as hostile take-overs and litigation. When, however, that line of business became vastly more important in the 1970s and afterwards, they were well-placed to dominate it (Fligstein, 2001: chs 6–7).

If we want to present this diagrammatically, we might do so through Figure 9.1. These contingent dynamics involve occupancy (of mainstream commercial law by Anglo-Saxon firms), closure (to Jewish entrants), eking out a survival on the margins (Jewish firms specialising in a low-regarded field), shifts in the commercial terrain (the sudden growth in hostile take-overs), new synergies (between corporates and the niche established by Jewish firms), a new terrain of their mutual advantage. In the language of Chapters 2 and 3, this is an evolutionary model of niche development and mutual adaptation, on a selective terrain which is itself shifting. In the language of Chapters 4 and 6, this is an account of agile action on complex terrains, shifting in response to larger structural changes that are under way.

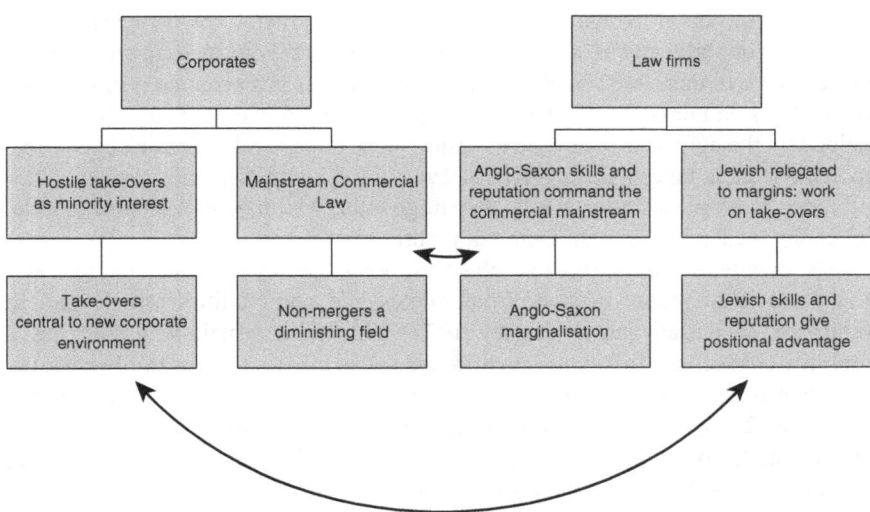

Figure 9.1 Success as cumulative contingency: law firms

It is not only Gladwell who identifies these dynamics – and the way that an innovation nurtured within a protected or marginal environment may then, when openings develop in the mainstream, flourish and even dominate. Christensen (2003: ch. 9) points out the difficulty that established industrial players find in developing innovations which lead in new directions ('disruptive technologies'). They typically need to establish a protected arena within which the potential of these innovations can be explored without regard to the settled ground of existing products. Only by this indirect route can established industrial players hope to probe new possibilities and progressively shift to new markets and value chains. Nevertheless, protection is not isolation: the innovator must stay sufficiently close to the big actors, to lever them in new directions (Gladwell, 2008: 139–51).

New openings do not always bring advance and success. A final case that Gladwell offers is the development of commercial aviation in Korea, one of the many new occupations that rapid industrialisation has brought (Gladwell, 2008: ch. 7). The settled knowledge and practices embedded in Korean society, which required deference towards seniors, meant that in the airplane cockpit the crew were unwilling to question the captain's decisions, even when these were liable to produce disaster. Korean airlines suffered very high levels of crashes. Only when aircrew were comprehensively retrained within an Anglo-Saxon culture of mutual criticism was the matter resolved. The settled knowledge and practices on which we draw, as we probe new opportunities, may be a recipe for success or disaster: that, too, is a matter of luck, although vigorous and deliberate action can then sometimes rework the situation.

Positional advantage and institutional careers

It would be possible to interpret what has been said so far as 'high rewards are a matter of luck'. That is not, however, what Gladwell is saying. From a public policy standpoint he is arguing for opportunities for all, so that we do not waste the talent and potential that arbitrary contingencies at present lead us to neglect. From the standpoint of individuals, he insists that while there is some element of luck, the lucky few still have to put in long hours of work and devotion, if they are to take advantage of the opportunity. There is, moreover, plenty of scope for them (and their parents) to create their own cumulative contingencies, to build their careers by shaping the institutional links around them, to build positional advantage for themselves and the organisations within which they work. To some degree we make our own good luck: and we make it by reworking the institutional rules, so that they are more likely to recognise our virtues, and to pardon our shortcomings.

The contingencies that really matter are those that link individual pathways to organisational success. It was because of major corporate changes under way in the 1970s that Jewish law firms expert in hostile take-overs were able to develop a new and strong niche; and it was because of the healthy state of Canadian ice hockey that youngsters who found themselves on an elite training programme were able to make this a prized and lucrative career. Getting selected for elite training, in a sport or skill that turns out to be an obsolete path to nowhere, will hardly seem like success.

It follows that any theory of high rewards that is rooted in this account of cumulative contingency will also be a theory of agile *career-building*. By this we mean a theory of how individuals *purposefully forge their own cumulative contingencies, so as to build positional advantage both for themselves and their organisations*. Success involves aligning your own future with that of the organisation: or else moving to an organisation where this will be possible. This is why the future direction of an organisation (in both senses of the word 'direction') commonly arouses such intense concern among its staff and its component units: and why they will compete and strive to shape that direction (Kristensen and Zeitlin, 2005). The ultimate prize is to ensure that the organisation and its directors recognise that they have arrived at a crucial moment and that you are one of the key players, in identifying the options before the organisation and implementing whichever is chosen. 'Cometh the hour, cometh the man or the woman': the right person in the right place at the right time. This is not in general a matter of luck, as it was with the birth month of Gladwell's young hockey players: it is an alignment which, to some degree, you have yourself brought to fruition.[6]

Success, therefore, means using Figure 9.1 – albeit in a more generic form – as the mental model of personal and organisational development; looking out for the points where crucial choices need to be made; and identifying the virtuous paths that can capture dynamic synergies, between your trajectory and that of your organisation. Here our discussion in Chapter 6 of the signs that social actors use to navigate such terrains may be apposite. It means identifying the capabilities that you and the organisation will need to acquire or develop – and which to abandon. It means standing back and arguing in terms that can have sufficiently broad appeal within the organisation. It is a matter not just of the technical skills you have developed, but of your rhetoric and leadership also.

A CEO needs to ensure that the organisation is one in which the right people are readily able to emerge with these visions: but not too readily, otherwise there will be a plethora of visions of little value. They need to be tested before they are brought into open debate. Such people are mission-critical, and the more complex and turbulent the environment, the more mission-critical they are.

Beyond luck

Gladwell's account of selection for the hockey elite has a larger import. The 'accident' of a birthday may determine whether young Canadians are offered elite training. More generally, however, the 'accident' of their parents' social class and ethnicity likewise shapes many of the other opportunities that come their way. Gladwell's conclusion, therefore, goes far beyond the world of hockey and team sports and asks why we waste so much talent and potential as a result of such arbitrary contingencies.

This raises major questions for public policy. It is easy to acknowledge that everyone should, in principle, continue their schooling for as long as they can benefit; and that this is most effectively and equitably judged by reference to their performance in the tests of performance that are set at each stage. Nevertheless, the result is that the distribution of educational investment across the population tends – at least beyond the school leaving age – to be very unequal. Against this, there is good evidence that, for a given financial outlay, it is investment in the lowest-skilled that can produce the greatest benefit, for national productivity at least (Coulombe *et al.*, 2004). There has also long been good evidence that positive discrimination in educational provision, targeting disadvantaged communities for additional school resources, can to some degree counter the wider inequalities that those children face (Halsey, 1972).

Gladwell's account of Jewish law firms also has larger import. Closed doors, he argues, can encourage the development of skills which in due course enable entry to newly emerging arenas. The particular example he chooses is one of racial discrimination, and it shows how those suffering such discrimination may eventually triumph. Nevertheless, Gladwell might struggle to find such cheering examples in the case of black – as distinct from Jewish – Americans.

Lieberson (1987) considers racial inequalities in the US, in schooling and in occupational destinations. Any success in reducing those educational inequalities is unlikely, he argues, to reduce corresponding inequalities in occupational outcomes, because more advantaged groups are likely to switch to other institutional means to maintain their position. This is a positional struggle, in which 'whites will give blacks as little as they can', consistent with the need 'to maintain the system and avoid having it overturned' (p. 191).

9.6 Agile leaders on complex terrains

We began this chapter with an explanation of rewards in terms of marginal products. Such explanations assume efficient markets, readily aligning the supply and demand for different skills. They also assume that the actors involved have sufficient information to make rational calculations, as to whether to train in particular skills for their future employment. This is a world that is stable, smoothly functioning and well-lit.

We have drawn on Gladwell's account of the accidents of birth, in relation to opportunities to train for elite hockey and other occupations. Nevertheless, as Gladwell recognises, the 'accidents' of birth that matter most are those associated with gender, race and class, and the advantages and disadvantages these entail. A few individuals from disadvantaged backgrounds may be lucky, and some from advantaged backgrounds unlucky: nevertheless, life chances in general depend on social background. As Goldthorpe and Breen argue, when young people from disadvantaged backgrounds consider whether to stay on at school, assessing the expected costs and benefits involved, they typically make the entirely rational decision that staying on makes little sense (Goldthorpe, 2007: ch. 3).

We also saw how the accident of birth into a Jewish family limited the opportunities within the legal profession, leaving Jewish lawyers to specialise in areas with few prospects. Gladwell does not record what happened to those rejected for elite hockey. He does tell us however about the larger changes in US corporate life that suddenly opened doors for the distinctive skills which Jewish lawyers had honed in their marginal niche. They now faced a whole new landscape, for which corporate America needed their skills and which those Jewish law firms could now colonise.

Thanks to the co-evolution of corporate America and these Jewish law firms, their niche now enjoyed vigorous new growth: low-hanging fruit which, for a time at least, they could expect to monopolise. This is just the sort of 'elective affinity' with which Chapter 3 dealt and which stood at the heart of our contingent historical model (CHM). The skills in which trainee Jewish lawyers had invested their time now appear in a new light, as compared with their original vocational calculation. However rational that calculation may have seemed at the time, job markets were wholly inadequate in signalling the supply and demand for different skills that those future co-evolutions were liable to produce.

The model with which we started – in terms of efficient markets, well-informed actors and marginal products – now seems clearly inadequate. Instead of social actors as *calculators of utility*, we require the very different model of social actors that we have developed in preceding chapters of this book: as *agile probers and re-weavers of their world* – endeavouring to discover and accelerate dynamic synergies around their specific capabilities and assets (see Chapters 3 and 4 above).

Rewards understood in terms of marginal products were not our only starting point. An alternative approach was concerned with rewards for risk-taking under conditions of dynamic and disruptive change. It pointed us to entrepreneurs and innovators, developing the technologies of the future, with some achieving market success, even if many others fail.

Nevertheless, we have also questioned this account of entrepreneurial risk-taking and the 'blind' processes by which the winners are selected. To start with, the larger the entrepreneur the more it is principally the capital of the shareholders that they risk (Fligstein, 2001: ch. 7). In addition, the larger the entrepreneur, the more likely they are to be able to shape the market, as market-makers rather than market-takers. 'Bounded rationality' is not evenly spread: the density of the fog varies. Those with power are better able to shape who sees what; information is asymmetric (Sayers, 2015: ch. 17). They may be able to perpetuate their gains by establishing intellectual property rights in the innovation: as for example with the modern pharmaceutical industry (Weiss *et al.*, 2004: ch. 5). They may be able to limit risk and the costs of uncertainty by displacing these onto others: albeit with disruption, for example, to the stable livelihoods of the company's workforce and the communities in which they live (Marris, 1982). The account of rewards for entrepreneurial risk-taking seems rather inadequate.

Instead we have suggested that our account of agile action offers a better vantage point from which to make sense of these leadership positions and the rewards that they command. This is 'leadership' exercised in relation to a complex and turbulent world of cumulative contingencies. After all, it is by reference to just such a notion of leadership that apologists for the modern corporate elite celebrate these 'masters of the universe' (Kapur et al., 2005; Soros, 2008): and that their arch-critics question their competence and denounce their predatory excesses (Peston, 2008; Brummer, 2009; Galbraith, 2009; Kay, 2009; Lankester, 2009; Tett, 2009; Treanor and Inman, 2009).[7]

What do leaders do?

Earlier chapters conceptualised agile action on complex terrains. This involved looking for points where crucial choices need to be made so as to capture dynamic synergies of transformational change. It involved using mental models to navigate such terrains and recognise turning points. It involved identifying the capabilities that an organisation will need to acquire or develop – and which ones to abandon. This is what Schön (1983) discusses in terms of 'reflection-in-action'.

What notion of leadership in action does this suggest: as the benchmark against which individual leaders might then reasonably be assessed?

Leaders survey possible futures for the threats and opportunities they may bring. They pool their insights and must collectively keep their nerve. They watch to see what dynamic synergies are forming, what emerging processes of self-organisation, such as those we discussed in Chapter 1. They watch for key turning points and they wait to intervene (Sayers, 2015: ch. 7).[8]

This requires the ability to acquire and evaluate real-time information as to what windows are opening or closing. It involves recognising and re-balancing risks, notwithstanding the complex interconnections that those risks involve (Blyth, 2013: ch. 2).

Leaders mobilise and combine, adapt and redeploy their organisation's capacities. It is this that Hirschman places at the centre of any strategic development process (Hirschman, 1958). This is *purposeful* action, involving negotiation, cooperation and imperative coordination.

They seek, to some degree, to align the organisation with the bigger actors shaping the terrain on which they find themselves. From this settled ground, leaders can assess the openings that are available for new initiatives; the fissures that might be exploited; the larger processes of structural change that are under way. This is what Chapter 8 discussed in terms of 'nuzzle'. From here they may be able to lever novel advantage and thereby dominate a larger expanse.

The complex dynamics of interconnected terrains make for a wide variety of possible futures: leaders do what they can to close down some possibilities and secure a preferred future. This will typically involve the building of alliances but also a contest between opposing visions of the future.

Such is the notion of leadership that apologists for the modern corporate elite celebrate and that accords with our own account of agile action. This is not all, however: and it is this that divides their apologists and their detractors. For the latter, what is no less the case is that many such leaders target windfalls – low-hanging fruit – which will afford easy pickings. This is wealth extraction rather than wealth creation. They multiply these windfalls by disrupting the institutional frameworks through which opportunities and rewards have hitherto been allocated. They offload risk and uncertainty onto others, the more to turn them into an opportunity for further predation (Galbraith, 2009). Under these conditions, those who secure high rewards do so largely as a form of institutionalised looting.[9]

How are leaders selected?

Leaders of organisations look out for individuals having the strategic know-how that is required in corporate strategy teams.[10] They judge between their different visions for the organisation's future. They recruit, induct and mentor their successors and separate them from more routine functions.

How is a CEO to recognise the rising talent – the mission-critical people – inside and outside the organisation? In many businesses, family, school and university connections play a part: and this may have had a certain justification, in ensuring a common culture and mutual trust within the corporate strategy group. More generally, they aim to admit and embrace the most capable and loyal of the upwardly mobile; and to bestow on them the appropriate wealth and style of life, not so much as a reward for effort, but to secure their moral commitment and loyalty. To use the distinction first made by Turner (1960), this is not so much 'contest mobility' as 'sponsored' mobility.

It is unsurprising then that, as Piketty (2014: 301) notes, the super-rich include several different social groups – some with very high incomes from inherited capital, others with high earned incomes – all united in defence and celebration of their shared position and accomplishments. After all, does not the wealth and privilege showered upon the super-managers, as marks of their success, demonstrate the efficiency with which the recruitment and promotion mechanisms of large corporations operate? This is what Weber discussed in terms of status group formation and closure (Gerth and Mills, 1948: ch. 7).

But what basis is there for confidence that these recruits are indeed the most capable of the upwardly mobile? As we have seen, Gladwell (2008) argues cogently that contingency – luck – is as important as talent, and that had chance produced a quite different set of candidates, a no less plausible celebration of their scarce talent would have emerged from the bosom of their new social home. To this extent, Piketty's 'meritocratic extremism' – the 'apparent need of modern societies to designate certain individuals as "winners"' (2014: 334) – reflects not so much the extraordinary talent of the beneficiaries, as the closure and solidarity of the various economic and political elites. This helps to ensure that few errors are made in selecting the members of these elites: or at least, few errors that cannot be kept decently invisible.

This solidarity, in turn, means separation from the wider society, with segregated arrangements for education, socialising and family formation and loss of any mutual sympathy (Dorling, 2014: chs 2, 4). These stand in sharp contrast to Tawney's advocacy – quoted in the previous chapter – of institutions which educate in civic concern and which 'emphasise and strengthen, not the class differences which divide, but the common humanity that unites' us (Tawney, 1931, 1964: 49).

How are leaders rewarded?

As we saw earlier, Avent-Holt and Tomaskovic-Devey (2013) argue that the process of reward determination is one of claim-making and negotiation. They have plenty to say about the rewards of the top earners in particular.

The latter typically claim that the organisation is in danger – or on the verge of a major breakthrough – and that their contribution at this particular juncture is critical. On the one hand, the corporate leadership promises to bring wealth from which all stakeholders in the organisation will benefit. On the other hand, loss of that leadership – for example if they are seduced by higher rewards elsewhere – may bring disaster. This is the argument for '*always keeping ahold of nurse, for fear of finding something worse*' (Belloc). This fear may be the more plausible, under conditions of disruption and turbulence.

It is also of course under these conditions that organisations may be especially vulnerable to predatory head-hunters, on the look-out for individuals with the strategic know-how that is developed in corporate strategy teams. Rival organisations may pay heavily for this: and for the disruption that any such departure will cause. How much should they pay? Is it a specific type of skill or contribution that is being hired and rewarded? Or is it indeed a matter of finding – and keeping ahold – of nurse? Is the role of such leaders simply to provide comfort against these existential fears, rather in the manner of the religious shaman, or indeed the teddy bear? Or maybe the better parallel is the medieval lord, the protector and guarantor against destruction, who in return is entitled to make off with all except the most basic means of livelihood.

The question remains: how much should they be paid? Today large organisations increasingly 'go with the crowd' on such matters: establishing remuneration committees and employing head-hunters who 'know the field'. These committees commonly have overlapping memberships drawn from the same social circles which bid up levels of pay (Hutton, 2015: ch. 4). The awards made by these committees also become means of signalling to rivals that this is a confident organisation: this may itself tend to reinforce upward pressure on already high rewards, with little or no justification (DiPrete *et al.*, 2010). Going with the crowd also tends to favour fashionable theories of executive skills: for example, the view that strategic corporate skills are generic, and that large banks for example can be run by people without banking experience.[11]

It should not, however, be assumed that where these judgements are misplaced, market pressures will over-ride them. On the contrary, Avent-Holt and Tomaskovic-Devey argue, they are often viable even in the long-term: 'Exploding executive pay can endure as other actors – workers and owners – are simply paid less' (2013: 388).

9.7 Conclusion

How shall we make sense of the growing levels of inequality within the countries of the western world? And what contribution can the perspectives developed in this book provide towards addressing that inequality?

Understanding inequality

Growing inequality in western societies has attracted plenty of attention, especially since the financial crisis of 2008. Until then it was possible to claim that wealth would 'trickle down' to the wider population: that claim has been viewed with increasing scepticism, as the costs of the 2008 crisis are visited on the wider population, even while a small elite continues to 'hoover up' a growing share of both income and wealth. International organisations such as the OECD, the IMF and the World Bank have joined the voices of alarm, pressing the case for 'shared prosperity' (World Bank, 2013).

This chapter has reconsidered the conventional explanations of unequal rewards but has found them wanting. It has, therefore, considered what light may be shed on the aforesaid inequalities by the account of complex and contingent dynamics offered in previous chapters, set within an understanding of political economy. In particular, it has argued that key aspects of income and wealth polarisation in the countries under review cannot be explained, without placing at the centre of attention the conjunctions of opportunities to make money with the capacity of the already wealthy to negotiate themselves into such situations.

In the late nineteenth century Pareto found that the upper levels of the distribution of income and wealth within advanced countries conformed to a 'power law' (Ball, 2004). Such power laws are the statistical 'signature' of complex dynamics and self-organising systems of the sort we introduced in Chapter 1. So are 'fat-tailed distributions' – in this case of income and wealth – which attest to the interconnections of different sorts of advantage, rather than their more random distribution across a population of representative individuals (Blyth, 2013: ch. 1; Sayer, 2015: 5–6). The very robustness of such distributions suggests that these inequalities are likely to be resilient in face of policy interventions.

It is worth considering the parallels with class inequalities in social mobility in advanced western societies. Goldthorpe's studies show that these have proved rather stable over much of the last hundred years (see Chapter 1 above). He points to pressures from those who are more advantaged, seeking to promote the life chances of their own children: these pressures would probably have exacerbated the inequalities in relative mobility chances, but for the social and educational policies of the post-war period, and the efforts of governments of different political hues to widen opportunity (Goldthorpe, 1980: 275; Erikson and Goldthorpe, 1993: 368). Here are two forms of agency, contesting the shifting terrain of educational opportunity. Room (2011b) has shown how this 'contingent' balance in social mobility is well captured by models drawn from the literature on complex systems: albeit understood by reference to the political economy of the societies in question.

In the present chapter we have found a rather different situation. Here, the pressures from the most advantaged have, in recent decades, met little or no countervailing and outflanking efforts from government. The cumulation of advantage, the disruption of established norms, the hollowing out of government and the weakening of trade unions leave little resistance to the self-aggrandisement of those who are lucky enough to find themselves blessed with windfalls. The contours of such a society, rather than being muted by 'push back', instead become ever starker.

But to what end? Why do people want to be so rich: and having become rich, why do they want to be even richer? Hacker and Pierson provide a clue. The efforts of the super-rich are devoted to 'shifting the risks of their new economic playground downward' (2010: 13). Amid the *anomie* and uncertainty of capitalist societies, the prize is to maintain freedom of manoeuvre, block unfavourable developments and offload uncertainty onto others (Marris, 1996; Pierson, 2004). This is a struggle to design and to 'occupy' the future: to ensure that come what may, tomorrow will turn out well (Sayer, 2015: 72, 79). This is why, as Keynes observes, the accumulation of wealth is often not so much for eventual consumption, it is for some indefinitely distant date, to ensure a place in the sun, whatever the future disposition of the world (Tily, 2007: 142). Not least, it assures the super-rich that come what may, their security and continued well-being will be assured.

Addressing inequality

This chapter has been argued in the shadow of the so-called Matthew principle:

> *For unto every one that hath shall be given, and he shall have abundance: but from him that hath not shall be taken away even that which he hath.*
> (Matthew 25:29)

What is the alternative? Maybe we should treat the leaders of large organisations as we do the captain of the ship or aircraft in which we are a passenger, or the surgeon or nursing staff who care for our loved ones: as responsible professionals who should expect a comfortable and respected lifestyle, but who should be ready to perform their roles as best they can, without demanding wealth beyond the dreams of avarice. This is what we might term the Luke principle:

> *For unto whomsoever much is given, of him shall be much required: and to whom men have committed much, of him they will ask the more.*
> (Luke 12:48)

This is consistent with the social contract suggested in the previous chapter, bringing all citizens together in a common endeavour (see also Hutton, 2015: 194ff.; Sayer, 2015: ch. 22).

Nevertheless, the prospects for such policies look rather poor. Especially in the US, the super-rich have benefitted over recent decades from the capital gains associated with neo-liberal deregulation and tax cuts. Such windfalls have enhanced their financial control of the major political parties. This political influence has enabled them to block social legislation and its application to the changing conditions of today's world (Hacker and Pierson, 2010: ch. 9; Sayers, 2015: ch. 15). In recent decades, it is from the rich and the major corporations that the most strident calls for protection of their interests have come, with government and the taxpayer underwriting the stability of the financial institutions in particular. With government-mandated pensions and government bonds increasingly mediated by those institutions, they simply cannot be allowed to fail. That gives them enormous leverage, politically as well as economically.

It may be difficult to reverse these pressures. The financial and institutional framework of our western societies – including in particular the US and the UK – has been re-woven and cannot be readily reworked. There are large swathes of our society who have lost out but there are many who to some degree have benefitted – and many more who are 'hunkered down' and would oppose any dramatic reforms, lest they find their situation only made worse (Sayer, 2015: 71, 202–4).

The negative consequences of the present situation are considerable.

First, the corrosive *anomie* of the economic system – reinforced by the super-rich, as they pursue the windfalls from which they derive their rewards – cannot be resolved by any self-equilibrating processes of the market system. It seems essential therefore that government – on behalf of the community as a whole – should be involved in reward determination, if only in terms of setting basic principles. Just as Keynes saw government as playing a key role in setting the investment climate and levels of business confidence in the economy, and just as Mazzucato insists that government has an indispensable role to play in developing enterprise and innovation, so we argue that it also has a necessary role to play in setting the framework within which rewards are determined and justified. This is consistent with the more general argument by Polanyi (1944) that markets and factors of production are socially and politically embedded.

Second, the cult of the super-hero, the CEO and the economic elite makes for a society which disregards the creativity of the citizenry – and indeed the workforce – at large. Contrast this with the argument in Chapter 8 for a social contract which invests in everyone's capabilities. This, we argued, is essential for securing public consent to change – but also for ensuring that the old and mature industrial economies of the west remain vibrant sources of creativity and enterprise, in face of the rising economic powers from the east. It is also important to recognise that enterprise and innovation benefit from the social and institutional contexts within which they develop and from many public policies, including on education, research and development, transport infrastructures, legal and commercial systems, etc. One corollary is that if enterprise and innovation presuppose a well-ordered society and a variety of public goods, for these the community is entitled to reap a dividend (Mazzucato, 2013; Sayer, 2015: ch. 9).

Third, extreme inequality puts environmental sustainability in question (Sayer, 2015: ch. 21). Recall Veblen's account of the 'leisure class' (Veblen, 1899). They advertise their success through their conspicuous consumption, which reinforces their social and economic distance from the larger society. This also provides ever-renewed symbols of the good life, to which that larger society is enjoined to aspire: the perennial creation of new consumption 'needs'. The race for ever-higher levels of personal consumption is less about meeting our needs, more about the race to keep up with unsustainable lifestyles, as a condition of social inclusion.

Social scientists are entitled – and are arguably under an obligation – to draw attention to these negative consequences, as a contribution to the social and political debate that is under way in the larger society. This requires them – as argued in Chapter 4 – to interrogate the super-rich as to the rationale for their actions. It also involves calling them to account for the way they exercise power (Lukes, 2005).

Economic orthodoxy, however, hardly acknowledges that economic actors do exercise power. They are individual actors responding to market signals. Whether we explain differential rewards by reference to marginal productivity or entrepreneurial risk, it is technologies and markets that matter and the choices that individuals make. Where there is no intention to coerce others, there can hardly be any exercise of power.

Hayward (2006) puts this in question. Even where there is no intention and even where individuals do not act collectively, it is reasonable to speak of their exercise of power and to assign responsibility for such negative consequences as those outlined above. In particular, she insists that this should apply not just to individuals but also to interconnected arrays or communities of actors whose actions impinge destructively on the interests of others.

She takes the example of 'middle-class flight' from inner-city areas. No one household can be said to be individually responsible for pushing the inner-city beyond some 'tipping point'; nevertheless, Hayward wants them to be held collectively to account for their restriction of the hopes and living conditions of their poorer neighbours. This argument resonates with that of Schelling (1978: ch. 4), discussed in Chapter 1. Starting with a random distribution of households across the city, Schelling shows that even a mild level of racial antipathy will quickly generate zones of racial segregation across the city. A parallel argument can be made about the activities of the super-rich and the corporate elites with whom the present chapter has been concerned (Room, 2015b).

Much of the world is non-linear; the effects of our individual actions may be counter-intuitive; the social scientist who can make sense of those non-linearities is better equipped to demonstrate these negative collective consequences of our individual actions and thereby to hold us collectively to account.[12] This, however, depends upon the theoretical paradigms and analytical tools of which the social scientist disposes. Complexity analysis can play a central and essential role in the analysis of power dynamics: and in revealing the emergent processes by which micro-behaviours – perhaps unwittingly – produce such destructive and cumulative effects. It must however be combined with political economy (Room, 2011a).

Notes

1 On the growing pay gap between corporate executives and their workforce, see www.theguardian.com/us-news/2015/aug/05/companies-disclosure-ceo-workforce-pay-gap.
2 Rather than the wage, it is more correct to say the net advantages of the job (Marshall, 1920: Book VI, chs 3–5).
3 It was in opposition to this that the Cambridge capital controversies of the 1960s and 1970s developed, questioning whether it was possible to speak in this way of the marginal product of capital (see, for example, Hahn and Matthews, 1965; Hunt and Schwartz, 1972).
4 The whole 'marginal principle' derives ultimately from Ricardo (1821). He, however, applied it to the different levels of productivity offered not by labour but by land. For Ricardo, rents resulted from established proprietorial rights: they rewarded past efforts, rather than today's toil. The 'marginal principle' was a means of analysing the monopoly element that such land ownership conferred, to the detriment of the truly productive sections of the population. Then as now, explanation was thus harnessed to normative criticism and calls for policy reform: landlords would not have accepted his analysis. In all this, the debate was primarily about who was entitled to take the *surplus*, once all 'necessary' costs of production had been met – and according to what institutional rules. On the contemporary relationship between entrepreneurs and rentiers see Dorling (2014: ch. 4) and Sayer (2015: Part 1).
5 For similar problems in British football, see www.bbc.co.uk/sport/olympics/18891749.
6 This is not limited to business elites. Similar processes operate in the public sector, including universities and the civil service (Stevens, 2011).
7 Within the management literature, writers such as Teece (2009) understand the sustainable advantage that enterprises enjoy in terms of the 'dynamic capabilities' that they bring together: all set within a co-evolutionary perspective on the business ecosystem. This is a perspective very similar to the account of agile action and positional advantage offered in preceding chapters of the present book.

It is also from this standpoint that Teece then identifies the key tasks of organisational leadership: and seeks to explain the high rewards that corporate leaders are paid (Teece, 2016). Nevertheless, this hardly accounts for the dramatic increases in such rewards, especially in the Anglo-Saxon countries, in recent years: indeed, in highlighting the skill with which they develop the businesses in question, it may also invite the question, as to whether they may not use those same skills to target the windfalls that such organisations generate and extract them for their own benefit.

Like much of the rest of the management literature, Teece does not differentiate between new technologies and products such as better mousetraps, and 'products' such as celebrity-style wedding packages and financial products of dubious provenance. The entrepreneurs in these latter cases are happy to expropriate the positive language of new technologies and new products, but the academic analyst needs to be suitably critical. At some point 'innovations' of this latter sort should arguably be couched in terms of predation: not value creation but value extraction. It is also surely necessary to understand these dynamic capabilities and sustainable advantage within the larger political economy and institutionalised arrangements for exercising power that operate in the countries concerned.
8 Other social scientists have similarly set such contingent variations within a historical setting: whether of individual social actors or of whole nations. Abbott (2001: ch. 8), for example, thinks of social actors and their life histories as a succession of choices at 'turning points': transitions which, he anticipates (p. 250), will typically be revealed by the changed significance or polarity of country-level variables, in national trajectories before and after the transition.
9 An obvious example is Goldman Sachs and their role in Greece's financial crisis: nations weakened by having to save their banks then become ideal targets for predatory

attack (Sayers, 2015: 210–11). A key element in these processes of wealth extraction has been the reordering and transformation of property relations including, for example, the privatisation of public assets and the demutualisation of building societies. These legal transformations – along with the definition of debtor and creditor relations – have been an integral part of the financial 'innovations' of recent decades.
10 Wake, in her history of the Kleinwort Benson Bank (1997: ch. 7), shows how just such a strategic dynamic dominated the company in the 1980s, as it readied itself to address the challenges and opportunities posed by the 'big bang' in the City of London.
11 The hapless Fred Goodwin, CEO at RBS, was an accountant, not a banker. At the end of 2015, a report by City regulators on HBOS and its collapse in 2008 raised major questions about the competence of its erstwhile senior executives: see www.theguardian.com/business/2015/nov/19/hbos-collapse-report-recommends-formal-investigation-into-former-executives.
12 Blyth (2013: 22) notes in reference to the financial crisis of 2008: 'What matters is how seemingly unconnected and opaque parts of the global system of finance came together to produce a crisis that none of those parts could have produced on its own ... the meltdown was a deeply non-linear and multi-causal process'.

References

Abbott, A. (2001), *Time Matters: On Theory and Method*, Chicago, IL: University of Chicago Press

Atkinson, A.B. (2015), *Inequality: What Can be Done?*, Cambridge, MA: Harvard University Press

Avent-Holt, D. and D. Tomaskovic-Devey (2013), 'A Relational Theory of Earnings Inequality', *American Behavioural Scientist* 58(3): 379–99

Ball, P. (2004), *Critical Mass: How One Thing Leads to Another*, London: Heinemann

Becker, G. (1964), *Human Capital: A Theoretical and Empirical Analysis with Special Reference to Education*, New York: Columbia University Press

Beinhocker, E.D. (2007), *The Origin of Wealth*, London: Random House

Bell, D. (1974), *The Coming of Post-Industrial Society*, London: Heinemann

Blau, P.M. and O.D. Duncan (1967), *The American Occupational Structure*, New York: Wiley

Blyth, M. (2013), *Austerity: The History of a Dangerous Idea*, New York: Oxford University Press

Brown, P., H. Lauder, and D. Ashton (2011), *The Global Auction*, Oxford: Oxford University Press

Brummer, A. (2009), *The Crunch: How Greed and Incompetence Sparked the Credit Crisis*, London: Random House

Brynjolfsson, E. and A. McAfee (2014), *The Second Machine Age*, New York: W.W. Norton

Christensen, C.M. (2003), *The Innovator's Dilemma*, New York: HarperCollins

Congressional Budget Office (2013), *The Distribution of Household Income and Federal Taxes, 2010*, Washington, DC: Congress of the United States

Coulombe, S., J.-F. Tremblay, and S. Marchand (2004), *Literacy Scores, Human Capital and Growth across Fourteen OECD Countries*, Ottawa: Statistics Canada

Crouch, C. (2011), *The Strange Non-Death of Neoliberalism*, Cambridge: Polity

DiPrete, T.A., G.M. Eirich, and M. Pittinsky (2010), 'Compensation Benchmarking, Leapfrogs and the Surge in Executive Pay', *American Journal of Sociology*, 115(6): 1671–712

Dorling, D. (2014), *Inequality and the 1%,* London: Verso

Erikson, R. and J.H. Goldthorpe (1993), *The Constant Flux: A Study of Class Mobility in Industrial Societies,* Oxford: Clarendon

Fligstein, N. (2001), *The Architecture of Markets: An Economic Sociology of Twenty-First Century Capitalist Societies,* Princeton, NJ: Princeton University Press

Frank, R. and P. Cook (1995), *The Winner-Take-All Society,* New York: Penguin

Galbraith, J.K. (2009), *The Predator State,* New York: Free Press

Gerth, H.H. and C.W. Mills (1948), *From Max Weber: Essays in Sociology,* London: Routledge

Gladwell, M. (2008), *Outliers: The Story of Success,* London: Penguin

Goldthorpe, J.H. (1974), 'Social Inequality and Social Integration in Modern Britain', in D. Wedderburn (ed.), *Poverty, Inequality and Class Structure,* Cambridge: Cambridge University Press: 217–34

Goldthorpe, J.H. (1978), 'The Current Inflation: Towards a Sociological Account', in F. Hirsch and J. H. Goldthorpe (eds), *The Political Economy of Inflation,* London: Martin Robertson: 186–216

Goldthorpe, J.H. (1980), *Social Mobility and Class Structure in Modern Britain,* Oxford: Clarendon Press

Goldthorpe, J.H. (1984), *Order and Conflict in Contemporary Capitalism,* Oxford: Oxford University Press

Goldthorpe, J.H. (1985), 'Problems of Political Economy after the End of the Post-War Period', in C. S. Maier (ed.), *Changing Boundaries of the Political,* Oxford: Oxford University Press: 363–407

Goldthorpe, J.H. (2007), *On Sociology (2nd edition): Volume Two: Illustrations and Retrospect,* Stanford, CA: Stanford University Press

Goldthorpe, J.H. and C. Mills (2008), 'Trends in Intergenerational Class Mobility in Modern Britain: Evidence from National Surveys, 1972–2005', *National Institute Economic Review,* 205: 83–100

Hacker, J.S. and P. Pierson (2010), *Winner-Take-All Politics,* New York: Simon and Schuster

Hahn, F.H. and R.C.O. Matthews (1965), 'The Theory of Economic Growth: A Survey', in American Economic Association and Royal Economic Society (ed.), *Surveys of Economic Theory,* London: Macmillan: 1–124

Halsey, A.H., (ed.) (1972), *Educational Priority: Volume 1: EPA Problems and Policies,* London: HMSO

Hayward, C.R. (2006), 'On Power and Responsibility', *Political Studies Review,* 4(2): 156–63

Hills, J., F. Bastagli, F. Cowell, H. Glennerster, E. Karagiannaki, and A. McKnight (2013), *Wealth in the UK: Distribution, Accumulation and Policy,* Oxford: Oxford University Press

Hirschman, A.O. (1958), *The Strategy of Economic Development,* New Haven, CT: Yale University Press

Hunt, E.K. and J.G. Schwartz (1972), *A Critique of Economic Theory,* Harmondsworth: Penguin

Hutton, W. (2015), *How Good We Can Be,* London: Little, Brown

Kapur, A., N. Macleod, and N. Singh (2005), *Plutonomy: Buying Luxury, Explaining Global Imbalances,* Citigroup. https://pissedoffwoman.wordpress.com/2012/04/12/the-plutonomy-reports-download/

Kay, J. (2009), 'What a Carve Up', *Financial Times,* 1 August

Keynes, J.M. (1936), *The General Theory of Employment, Interest and Money,* London: Macmillan

Kristensen, P.H. and J. Zeitlin (2005), *Local Players in Global Games: The Strategic Constitution of a Multinational Corporation*, Oxford: Oxford University Press

Lankester, T. (2009), 'The Banking Crisis and Inequality', *World Economics*, 10(1): 151–6

Lieberson, S. (1987), *Making it Count: The Improvement of Social Research and Theory*, Berkeley: University of California Press

Lukes, S.M. (2005), *Power: A Radical View (Second Edition)*, Basingstoke: Palgrave Macmillan

Lundvall, B.-A., P. Intarakumnerd, and J. Vang, (eds) (2006), *Asia's Innovation Systems in Transition*, Cheltenham: Edward Elgar

Marris, P. (1982), *Community Planning and Conceptions of Change*, London: Routledge and Kegan Paul

Marris, P. (1996), *The Politics of Uncertainty*, London: Routledge

Marshall, A. (1920), *Principles of Economics*, London: Macmillan

Mazzucato, M. (2013), *The Entrepreneurial State*, London: Anthem

Mincer, J. (1974), *Schooling, Experience and Earnings*, New York: Columbia University Press

Peston, R. (2008), *Who Runs Britain?* London: Hodder and Stoughton

Pierson, P. (2004), *Politics in Time*, Princeton, NJ: Princeton University Press

Piketty, T. (2014), *Capital in the Twenty-First Century*, Cambridge, MA: Belknap/Harvard University Press

Polanyi, K. (1944), *The Great Transformation*, New York: Rinehart

Potts, J. (2000), *The New Evolutionary Microeconomics: Complexity, Competence and Adaptive Behaviour*, Cheltenham: Edward Elgar

Ricardo, D. (1821), *Principles of Political Economy and Taxation*, London: John Murray

Rogers, E. (2003), *Diffusion of Innovations*, New York: Simon and Schuster, 5th edition

Room, G. (2011a), *Complexity, Institutions and Public Policy: Agile Decision-Making in a Turbulent World*, Cheltenham: Edward Elgar

Room, G. (2011b), 'Social Mobility and Complexity Theory: Towards a Critique of the Sociological Mainstream', *Policy Studies*, 32(2): 109–26

Room, G. (2015a), 'Capital, Inequality and Public Policy', *Journal of European Social Policy* 25(2): 242–8

Room, G. (2015b), 'Complexity, Power and Policy', in R. Geyer and P. Cairney (eds), *Handbook on Complexity and Public Policy*, Cheltenham: Edward Elgar

Sayer, A. (2015), *Why We Can't Afford the Rich*, Bristol: Policy Press

Schelling, T.C. (1978), *Micromotives and Macrobehaviour*, London: W.W. Norton

Schön, D.A. (1983), *The Reflective Practitioner*, New York: Basic Books

Smith, Y. (2010), *Econned*, London: Palgrave Macmillan

Soros, G. (2008), *The New Paradigm for Financial Markets*, London: Perseus Books

Stevens, A. (2011), 'Telling Policy Stories: An Ethnographic Study of the Use of Evidence in Policy-Making in the UK', *Journal of Social Policy*, 40(02): 237–55

Tawney, R.H. (1931, 1964), *Equality*, London: Unwin Books

Teece, D.J. (2009), *Dynamic Capabilities and Strategic Management*, Oxford: Oxford University Press

Teece, D.J. (2016), 'Dynamic Capabilities and Entrepreneurial Management in Large Organizations: Toward a Theory of the (Entrepreneurial) Firm', *European Economic Review*. http://dx.doi.org/10.1016/j.euroecorev.2015.11.006

Tett, G. (2009), *Fool's Gold*, London: Little, Brown

Tily, G. (2007), *Keynes's General Theory, The Rate of Interest and 'Keynesian' Economics: Keynes Betrayed*, London: Palgrave Macmillan

Toner, P. (1999), *Main Currents in Cumulative Causation: The Dynamics of Growth and Development,* London: St Martin's Press

Treanor, J. and P. Inman (2009), 'Business as Usual for the Bankers', *Guardian,* 4 August

Turner, R.H. (1960), 'Sponsored and Contest Mobility and the School System', *American Sociological Review,* 25(6): 855–62

Veblen, T. (1899), *The Theory of the Leisure Class,* New York: Macmillan

Wagener, H.-J. and J.W. Drukker, (eds) (1986), *The Economic Law of Motion of Modern Society: A Marx-Keynes-Schumpeter Centennial,* Cambridge: Cambridge University Press

Wake, J. (1997), *Kleinwort Benson: The History of Two Families in Banking,* Oxford: Oxford University Press

Weiss, L., E. Thurbon, and J. Mathews (2004), *How to Kill a Country: Australia's Devastating Trade Deal with the US,* Crows Nest: Allen and Unwin

Wootton, B. (1955), *The Social Foundations of Wages Policy,* London: George Allen and Unwin

World Bank (2013), *Inclusion Matters: The Foundation for Shared Prosperity,* Washington, DC: World Bank

Conclusion

This book has been concerned with public policy and the social science on which it draws. More specifically, it has been concerned with complex and non-linear policy terrains, the positional struggles which unfold upon them and the scope for wise and reasonable public policies. This conclusion sums up some of the insights that have emerged, in terms of understanding these terrains and guiding action.

Understanding complex terrains

The foregoing chapters have addressed some significant questions in social theory and the methodology of the social sciences. These include the role and the limitations of linear models; complex systems and the emergence of order; agile action and its relationship to habitual and rational action; realist philosophies of social science. These disputes within the academy are not without consequence for the world of policy and practice – not least via our training of students who move into that real world and must make of it what they can.

Should we view that world as a set of discrete problems, the solutions to which can be tested and compared as though in a laboratory, with its canons of controlled experimentation? Or should we start from the assumption that the social world is highly interconnected, a dense and dynamic ecosystem, where little can be said about one bit without also saying something about the whole? That holistic vision is compelling – but it may also discourage us from venturing more modest and delimited conclusions about the world taken in bite-sized chunks. The better question may, therefore, be: when and under what conditions should we view the world in these two different ways?

We have argued that it is possible to develop an analytical perspective on this social world of dynamic interconnections: but that not enough effort has gone into developing such tools, relative to the efforts made with linear models. The latter may be an appropriate starting point for the training of our students, as future policy analysts and policy-makers, but they are not sufficient.

Our conclusion in regards to the complexity literature and its relevance to the social world can be simply stated. Its vision of a dynamically connected world is fruitful and enlightening, as are the various forms of 'self-organisation' to which it points: but only if we also recognise the struggle for positional advantage in which social actors are involved, the contested institutional tools of that struggle and the encompassing political economy. Such a dynamic perspective thus sits comfortably with other major concerns of the social science community, notably in regards to the contestation of institutional arrangements and the exercise of power within our societies.

The complexity literature, coming largely from the natural and informational sciences, encourages us to think in new ways about the social world. It challenges our intuitions and our taken-for-granted ways of approaching our subject matter:

- It re-trains us to think in terms of *open* and not just *closed* systems: systems that are variously connected to their larger environment.
- It makes us think in terms of the potential non-linear and counter-intuitive consequences of a micro-change, depending upon the dynamic synergies that this micro-change develops with other elements of the system.
- It tells us that rather than thinking of systems that tend towards equilibrium, we should expect them to exhibit quite different sorts of dynamic behaviour, depending on the underlying parameters and connections of the system in question.
- It tells us that even the most stable ground may over time move towards a *bifurcation* (or 'tipping') point, shifting to a new configuration or becoming unstable and even collapsing altogether.

This reading of the complexity literature is common to a wide range of scholars who have sought to apply its insights to the social world. Where the present book and its predecessor (Room, 2011a) are perhaps somewhat distinctive is in the combination that they build between complexity and the institutionalist and political economy literatures. It is by nurturing this synthesis that we seek to exploit the synergies – the elective affinities – between these different intellectual currents.

The foregoing chapters show how this can be done. For example, as we saw in Chapter 1, Lieberson and Goldthorpe offer similar accounts of the race between government taking measures to promote equality, and more advantaged families seeking to defend and reinforce their positions (Lieberson, 1987; Erikson and Goldthorpe, 1993: 368–9, 393–7). This cannot be modelled as an equilibrium: for 'no equilibrium is really possible between the different causal forces' (Lieberson, 1987: 190). What seems much more appropriate is the sort of model that Bak offers, in terms of 'punctuated equilibrium' and 'self-organised criticality' (Bak, 1997). Formal models of such dynamics are widely developed within the complexity literature: their application to the sort of empirically oriented sociology represented by Lieberson and Goldthorpe is long overdue (Room, 2011b).

Chapter 3 referred to the work of policy scientists who have been inspired by evolutionary perspectives on change, including Thelen (2004) and Palier (2010): both concerned to understand institutional change and the purposive struggles involved. It also referred to Esping-Andersen (1990): examining the struggles between different social classes around welfare systems and social policies.

Nevertheless, neither Esping-Andersen nor Thelen offer any formal models or tools that can bring analytical leverage to this history, allowing them to confirm, beyond the limited range of countries they study, the processes of evolution and lock-in that they infer. We argued therefore for the 'marriage' of these 'thick' qualitative and historical accounts with the formal analytic developed in Chapter 3 from the work of Jain and Krishna (2003): an analytic that arises from the rich literature on co-evolutionary dynamics that is now available (Crutchfield and Schuster, 2003; Solé and Bascompte, 2006).

Both of these examples show how a complexity perspective and the non-linear models that it brings can enrich institutionally grounded social science. Such a social science can in turn provide a vantage point for reconsidering some of the standard models used by complexity pioneers. Recall for example the model of residential segregation used by Schelling (1978), to which several of our chapters have referred. He posits a 'tolerance schedule', a preference not to have within one's immediate neighbourhood more than a certain proportion of another race. Through repeated simulations, he shows that even a rather mild level of racial antipathy will quickly generate zones of racial segregation across the city. Such individual preferences are, in reality, more plastic and multi-dimensional than his model suggests. Moreover, far from being a given, they are in considerable part formed by the institutional dynamics in which social actors find themselves and the insecurities to which they are exposed. The latter are, in turn, shaped to some degree by the public policies of the day and the menu of choices these make available to individual households (Room, 2011a: ch. 15). To repeat, therefore: in using the models of non-linear dynamics provided by the complexity literature, social scientists must have due regard to the institutional contexts.

The General Linear Model (GLM) has long exerted a powerful and seductive sway across the social sciences. Its critics have therefore had an uphill task. They have largely failed to develop an alternative in terms which can match the attractions of the GLM: its ease of visualisation, its formalisation in terms of simple equations, its convenience and tractability.[1]

Many of those inspired by the complexity literature to develop such a critique have done so by skilful computational modelling of non-linear dynamics (including but not confined to agent-based modelling). The results exhibit a degree of technical sophistication that can match that of the exponents of the GLM. As we noted in Chapter 1, however, those who have elaborated computational models often fail to ground them empirically; and such models typically have little to say about the institutional and political settings within which these non-linear effects emerge (Boero and Squazzoni, 2005; Room, 2011a: ch. 13; Byrne and Callaghan, 2014: ch. 7).

It is for this reason that Chapter 3 developed our Contingent Historical Model (CHM) of co-evolutionary dynamics, in a form that is easy to visualise, susceptible to formal modelling, empirically applicable and usable in conjunction with 'thick' qualitative accounts of positional struggle within specific institutionalist and political economy contexts. To develop such a synthesis has been one of the primary concerns of this book.

Acting on complex terrains

A second concern has been with the implications for social action and public policy: and for the part that social science can play, in illuminating the policy world and ensuring a 'well-conducted critical discussion' of our public affairs (Popper, 1994) (see also Chapter 4 above).

We have argued for a continuing 'dance' between the self-organisation that may 'emerge' and, on the other hand, the efforts of policy-makers – and other actors – to impose organisation and strategic direction of their own. It is folly to suggest that society self-organises without reference to the distribution of power – or that the market, left to itself, can achieve this magic. Leaving the market to itself is a specific choice on behalf of the society in which we live – a choice which is likely to play to the interests of those with market power.

If – whether as scholars or as citizens – we reject that choice, we are entitled to ask about other forms of self-organisation and political direction. Here we may, for example, appeal to traditions of social democracy and look to government for benign, wise, competent and far-sighted stewardship of the common weal. In an earlier generation that hope was shared in their different ways by Keynes and Beveridge, Roosevelt and J.K. Galbraith. How well in practice governments can meet such high ambitions is, however, quite another matter: the same goes for the various social movements aiming to promote the public good.

We have argued for active government to steer the dynamic and interconnected system that provides each of us with some stable and settled ground. Only on such a condition can most of us hope to develop our creative capacities, contribute to the production and reproduction demands of our communities and hold power to account. Even so, there will be some who withdraw from this common endeavour, even while they predate on the wealth that it produces, destabilising the stable ground on which the rest of us depend. Central to this insecurity is the cultural and economic power of the super-rich – what Veblen (1899) described as the 'leisure class'. That is why the active and countervailing involvement of the mass of citizens in the business of government is necessary for a civilised order.

We have tended to emphasise those policy interventions that set new dynamic synergies in train (see, for example, Chapter 7 above). There is also, however, the intervention that simplifies those connections and pursues a course of 'de-complexity' (Stewart, 2001, 2003). One obvious example again is provided by the financial crisis that began in 2008. This arose in part from the high level of coupling across the financial system. This has led to proposals for separating 'retail' and 'investment' banks, with more buffers or 'firebreaks', so as to ensure greater resilience and robustness (Kay, 2009).

The individual bankers did not and could not see to what systemic problems their actions would collectively give rise. One of the tasks of the social researcher is to illuminate these non-linear and counter-intuitive consequences, to interrogate the unwitting instigators and to hold them to account (Hayward, 2006). A second task is to map the alternative institutional rules which would mitigate those effects: albeit no rules will suffice, without regulatory oversight and occasional further intervention, to promote and protect the public interest. A third task is to illuminate and inform the deliberative democracy by which citizens at large can join in defining and defending that public interest.

This presupposes – to some degree at least – a cohesive national community and civic bodies that can watch and act on behalf of the public good. There are, however, limitations to what public policy can achieve within the confines of individual nations. This is in part because the policy terrains with which national policy-makers deal are, to varying degrees, trans- and supra-national, requiring a concerted approach. It is also because those terrains are dominated by corporate actors, skilled in playing off national authorities against each other (Blyth, 2013: ch. 1).

Imperial rulers systematically extracted wealth from the colonies they governed, with little if any regard for the welfare of the peoples in question. As the corporate rich organise themselves across national boundaries, it may be more appropriate to make sense of their power and privileges, not as fellow members of our national communities, but as just such an occupying power. They are after all increasingly removing themselves – physically, legally and politically – from the national communities in which the rest of us live: dissociating themselves from the ties and obligations of such a community (Piketty, 2014: 464–5). It is hardly possible for them to be held to account.

It may be that our national traditions of democratic debate – and indeed the traditions of intellectual discussion in the academy – have left us disabled from posing such issues. We take for granted that within such national and intellectual communities, it should be possible to analyse social arrangements and distributions by reference to shared standards of individual worth and rational debate. In the words of Popper, we expect a 'well-conducted critical discussion', in which we can debate the rationale and justification for these social arrangements (see Chapter 4 above). That may be an illusion.

Making things simple

This book began on the hillsides of Svalbard. It described how self-organisation of the hillside developed – but also how this 'simplified' the escarpment. The discussion through subsequent chapters may at times have been somewhat demanding, for reader as much as for writer, but the policy message with which the book concludes is likewise rather simple.

In the introductory chapter we referred to 'wicked' problems. Complex dynamics can produce a tangled knot of institutions and policy interventions, with path dependencies and lock-ins which are hard to escape, and trade-offs which allow of no easy resolution. This book suggests that such problems are unlikely to be solved by leaving them to the market, or by improving the technical skills of those in government. What is needed instead is the distributed intelligence and wisdom of all those involved and cooperative solutions: moving the system towards an alternative dynamic.

What alternative dynamics might this entail? The literature on complex systems emphasises that quite small changes in initial conditions can result in dramatically different dynamics and directions of travel (Kauffman, 2008). It underlines that the future is open: there is *always* an alternative. This chimes well with longstanding critiques of 'futurology' (Goldthorpe, 1972). Nevertheless, faced with an open future, the more powerful do not hesitate to intervene, to ensure as far as possible that their interests are protected, their position consolidated and the costs of uncertainty displaced onto others. This is what in earlier chapters we referred to as 'occupying the future'.

One of the tasks of the social scientist is to expose how these powerful groups narrow the range of possible futures. A second is to illuminate other possible paths of development, thereby enriching democratic debate. This is no merely technical matter. After all, these alternative futures span the different values by which citizens live their lives and express their hopes and their fears (Scott, 1998: ch. 10; Klein, 2007: Conclusion; Coleman, 2014: Conclusion).

What of our political leaders? How should they act and what can we hope for from them? Lukes argues for 'forward-looking' responsibility on the part of 'politically responsible agents, in strategic positions, who are able to make a difference' (Lukes, 2006: 172). The content that policy-makers give to this will depend on how they see their fellow citizens. Rational action theories taken from the academy into the policy realm encourage them to think of those citizens as competitive consumers in search of multiple choices. Behavioural approaches encourage a focus on their inertia, their risk aversion and their biases.

Our own approach, in terms of agile action on complex terrains, suggests a different policy vision altogether (see also the social contract discussed in Chapter 8). It is necessary, first, for public policy to ensure solidarity and compensation across the society as a whole, if the damages produced by urban-industrial change are not to lie where they fall. This was a central argument by Titmuss, perhaps the most authoritative of the post-war generation of scholars who mapped the contours of social policy (Titmuss, 1968: ch. 11). Building security for the mass of the population also limits opportunities for the financial sector to make money by predatory activities (Galbraith, 2009).

It also involves active management of the economy as a complex system. This includes ambitious programmes of social investment, so as to maximise creative potential across the society. Policies of austerity which prescribe withdrawal of government from the self-organising market are the enemy of innovation and growth (Blyth, 2013; Mazzucato, 2013; Room, 2015).

It is from this vantage point – alongside its rivals – that we can hope to inspire and train our students, as the new generation of agile policy-makers, in what will doubtless remain a complex and turbulent world.

Note

1 This is not the only case in scientific development where mathematical sophistication and self-assurance have overwhelmed the doubters and where epistemological technique has been used to conceal ontological weakness. Colander and Kupers (2014: ch. 10) and Bliss (2010) both highlight the failure of the opponents of economic

orthodoxy during the post-war decades to provide a sufficiently robust mathematical vindication of their alternative. Colander and Kupers add (ch. 9) that this allowed the orthodox to define the disagreement as one just of epistemological technique, deflecting challenges to their own ontological foundations.

References

Bak, P. (1997), *How Nature Works: The Science of Self-Organized Criticality,* Oxford: Oxford University Press

Bliss, C. (2010), 'The Cambridge Post-Keynesians: An Outsider's Insider View', *History of Political Economy,* 42(4): 631–52. doi: 10.1215/00182702-2010-031

Blyth, M. (2013), *Austerity: The History of a Dangerous Idea,* New York: Oxford University Press

Boero, R. and F. Squazzoni (2005), 'Does Empirical Embeddedness Matter? Methodological Issues on Agent-Based Models for Analytical Social Science', *Journal of Artificial Societies and Social Simulation,* 8(4). http://jasss.soc.surrey.ac.uk/8/4/6.html

Byrne, D. and G. Callaghan (2014), *Complexity Theory and the Social Sciences,* Abingdon: Routledge

Colander, D. and R. Kupers (2014), *Complexity and the Art of Public Policy,* Princeton, NJ: Princeton University Press

Coleman, G. (2014), *Hacker, Hoaxer, Whistleblower, Spy: The Many Faces of Anonymous,* London: Verso

Crutchfield, J.P. and P. Schuster, (eds) (2003), *Evolutionary Dynamics,* Oxford: Oxford University Press

Erikson, R. and J.H. Goldthorpe (1993), *The Constant Flux: A Study of Class Mobility in Industrial Societies,* Oxford: Clarendon

Esping-Andersen, G. (1990), *The Three Worlds of Welfare Capitalism,* Cambridge: Polity Press

Galbraith, J.K. (2009), *The Predator State,* New York: Free Press

Goldthorpe, J.H. (1972), 'Theories of Industrial Society: Reflections on the Recrudescence of Historicism and the Future of Futurology', *European Journal of Sociology,* 12: 263–88

Hayward, C.R. (2006), 'On Power and Responsibility', *Political Studies Review,* 4(2): 156–63

Jain, S. and S. Krishna (2003), 'Graph Theory and the Evolution of Autocatalytic Networks', in S. Bornholdt and H.G. Schuster (eds), *Handbook of Graphs and Networks,* Weinheim: Wiley-VCH: 355–95

Kauffman, S.A. (2008), *Reinventing the Sacred: A New View of Science, Reason and Religion,* New York: Basic Books

Kay, J. (2009), *Narrow Banking: The Reform of Banking Regulation,* London: Centre for the Study of Financial Innovation

Klein, N. (2007), *The Shock Doctrine,* London: Penguin

Lieberson, S. (1987), *Making it Count: The Improvement of Social Research and Theory,* Berkeley: University of California Press

Lukes, S.M. (2006), 'Reply to Comments', *Political Studies Review,* 4(2): 164–73

Mazzucato, M. (2013), *The Entrepreneurial State,* London: Anthem

Palier, B., (ed.) (2010), *A Long Goodbye to Bismarck? The Politics of Welfare Reform in Continental Europe,* Amsterdam: Amsterdam University Press

Piketty, T. (2014), *Capital in the Twenty-First Century,* Cambridge, MA: Belknap/Harvard University Press

Popper, K.R. (1994), 'Models, Instruments and Truth: The Status of the Rationality Principle in the Social Sciences', in K.R. Popper (ed.), *The Myth of the Framework: In Defence of Science and Rationality,* London: Routledge: 154–84

Room, G. (2011a), *Complexity, Institutions and Public Policy: Agile Decision-Making in a Turbulent World,* Cheltenham: Edward Elgar

Room, G. (2011b), 'Social Mobility and Complexity Theory: Towards a Critique of the Sociological Mainstream', *Policy Studies,* 32(2): 109–26

Room, G., (ed.) (2015), *Alternatives to Austerity,* Bath: Institute for Policy Research, University of Bath

Schelling, T.C. (1978), *Micromotives and Macrobehaviour,* London: W.W. Norton

Scott, J.C. (1998), *Seeing like a State,* Newhaven, CT: Yale University Press

Solé, R. and J. Bascompte (2006), *Self-Organization in Complex Ecosystems,* Princeton, NJ: Princeton University Press

Stewart, M. (2001), *The Coevolving Organization: Poised between Order and Chaos,* Rutland: Decomplexity Associates. www.decomplexity.com/

Stewart, M. (2003), *The Robust Organization: Highly Optimised Tolerance,* Rutland: Decomplexity Associates. www.decomplexity.com/

Thelen, K. (2004), *How Institutions Evolve,* Cambridge: Cambridge University Press

Titmuss, R.M. (1968), *Commitment to Welfare,* London: Unwin

Veblen, T. (1899), *The Theory of the Leisure Class,* New York: Macmillan

Index

Abbott, A. 18, 51, 52–3, 54, 71n5, 101, 184n8
access 97
accountability 89
ACS *see* autocatalytic sets
action theory 83–5
active citizenship 146; action in face of uncertainty 149–51; budge 147–9, 157, 158n5, 159n8; nudge 146–7, 148, 149, 150, 153, 158n5; nuzzle 151–3, 154, 158n5, policy nuzzles 153–5; conclusion 155–8
adaptive walks 103, 113
advantage 94, 95, 101; *see also* positional advantage
adverse incorporation 44
Affluent Worker studies 91n16, 117
agent-based modelling 15–16
agile action 35–8, 81–3, 88–9, 90n10, 91n12, 110, 151, 159n10; and the rationale of institutions 85–8
agile actors 2–3
agile leaders on complex terrains 175–7; leadership 177–8; rewards for leaders 179; selection of leaders 178–9
agile opportunism and 'luck' 171
agile probing for positional advantage 112–14, 176
alignments 115, 121n10
Allen, P. 18
'animal spirits' of capitalists 167
anomalous patterns 37
anomie 100, 106, 169–70, 182
Anonymous hackers 91n17
anthropogenic change 34, 46n5
Archer, M.S. 91n12

Arthur, W.B. 159n12
artificial selection 33, 35, 39, 42, 44, 66
arts of civilisation 32, 34, 39–40; and the Contingent Historical Model 60, 61–2
Atkinson, A.B. 164
Australasia 56, 57
autocatalytic sets (ACS) 64–6, 65*f*
autonomous social, economic and political hinterlands 98
Avent-Holt, D 169, 179

'backward-looking' attribution of blame 89
Bak, P. 21, 24
balanced growth 20
Ball, P. 16
Bayesian search and decision process 113, 121n6
Behavioural Insights Unit 127, 154
behaviourism 2
Beinhocker, E.D. 47n10, 167
Belloc, H. 179
Benington, J. *et al.* 141
Bevan, P. 95, 101
bifurcations 15, 24
big actors 87–8, 114, 151–2, 153, 156, 157, 159–60n13, 160n21
big data 25, 66, 119
biological selection 32, 46n2
Bliss, C. 194–5n1
Blyth, M. 118, 180, 183
Boero, R. 25
Boolean algebra 72n10
bounded rationality 111–12, 176
Bourdieu, P. 91n12, 107n5–6
Breakwell, G.M. 116

Bronowski, J. 16, 46n4
Brown, G. 53
Brown, P. et al. 107n2
Brynjolffson, E.J. et al. 87, 168
budge 147–9, 157, 158n5, 159n8
Burt, R.S. 97–8, 105, 112, 159n13
Byrne, D. 72n10, 143n7

calculators of utility 83, 85, 91n13, 176
Campbell Collaboration 127–8
Campbell, D.T. 15, 119, 127–8, 129, 137
capitalism 19, 90n8, 152, 156, 164, 167
capitalist accumulation 167
career-building 174
causal chains 41
causal powers 22
CDP see Community Development Project
CHM see Contingent Historical Model
choice architecture 106, 147; see also positional advantage
Christakis, N. 114
Christensen, C.M. 97, 114, 173
Chung, H. 159n6
citizenship 45–6
City of London 185n10
Clark, T. 159n6
closed systems 52
co-evolution 58, 133
Coalition Government 127, 149
Cochrane Collaboration 127, 142n5
Colander, D. 194–5n1
Coleman, G. 87, 91n17
Coleman, J. 15
collective responsibility 106
Collingwood, R.G. 89n1
combinatorial ontology 39, 61
common pool resources 86
Community Development Project (CDP) 53, 140–2
complex terrains 189–91; acting on complex terrains 192–3; see also navigating complex environments
complexity 3, 5, 183, 190
complexity and the social sciences: emergence of order 9–12; self-organisation and the imposition of order 19–21; social emergence 12–19; transformative realism 21–6; conclusion 26

computational simulation 25
connections across boundaries 97–8
Conservative Government 127, 149
conspicuous consumption 43, 155, 160n18
contingent development 50; evolution as contingent development 55–7, 104; General Linear Model 50–1, 51f; limitations of the GLM 51–5; conclusion 68–70; see also Contingent Historical Model
Contingent Historical Model (CHM) 57–60, 58f, 60f; and the arts of civilisation 60, 61–2; methodological implications 62: (autocatalytic sets 64–6, 65f; purposive struggles 66–8; qualitative system dynamics 62–4, 63f); conclusion 68–70
'control parameters' 15, 24
conventions see habits and conventions
cooperation 87, 95
corporate elite 166
counter-intuitive patterns 90n11
Court, J. 130
Coventry CDP 141–2
creative destruction 167
critical discussion 78
critical path analysis 20
Crouch, C. 17, 39, 61, 90n10, 150
cumulative causation 40, 71n8

Dahl, R.A. 102
Darwin, C. 3, 11, 31–2, 34, 40, 46n3, 46n4, 55, 132–3; Tree of Life 56, 56f, 57–8, 64, 65, 132, 133f
Darwin, J. 98, 101, 115, 152–3
Dawe, A. 13, 16, 17, 41, 85, 95
Dawkins, R. 32
Deák, I. et al. 87, 101
decent jobs 156
decision-theoretic framework 90n6, 121n3
deliberative democracy 157–8
Desai, M. 19
disruptive technologies 114
distributed intelligence 87, 172
'distributed systems' 18
Dopfer, K. 13
Dorling, D. 164
Dowling, C. 121n7
Downing Street 'Nudge Unit' 154

'downward causation' 15, 23
Durkheim, E. 13, 27n8, 100
dynamic capabilities 184n7

EBPM *see* evidence-based policy-making
economic development 19–20
economic policy 45
ecosystems 13
education 96, 107n2, 149–50, 171, 175
Educational Priority Area programme (EPA) 140
Elder-Vass, D. 27n8, 27n10
Eldridge, N. 40
elective affinity 59, 68, 71n4, 81, 176
emergence 3
entrepreneurial activity 17, 61–2
entrepreneurial state 167
entrepreneurs 39
entropy 26n3
Eppel, E. *et al.* 114, 119, 120, 121n8
equilibrium 13, 31, 40, 44
Esping-Andersen, G. 67, 156
Etzioni, A. 24, 86
evidence-based policy-making (EBPM) 22, 127–8, 142n2; as the assessment of impact 128–30, 129f, 130f; the case for transformative realism 132–6, 133f, 135f, 143n9–10: (case study 140–2, 143n11); choosing a paradigm 136–7, 136f; the ontological challenge of realism 130–2, 132f, 143n6–7; protocols for evidence 138–9; conclusion 137
evolution 103; as contingent development 55–7, 104; path-dependency 38–9, 47n10, 55–6, 104; *see also* fitness
evolution and the arts of civilisation 31; agile action 35–8; combinatorial contingency: unlocking potential 38–41; Darwin's journey reversed 31–5; policy science 44–6; positional struggle 41–4
evolutionarily stable state 60
evolutionary version *see* transformative realism
exclusion 97

'fast' and 'slow' thinking 111–12, 116, 150
fat-tailed distributions 180
first mover advantage 99, 159n12, 168

Fisher, L. 117
Fisher, R.A. 107n7
fitness 41–2, 103, 104, 105
fitness landscapes 38–9, 38f, 40, 55, 107n7; and positional advantage 103–5, 103f, 113; rugged landscape 103f, 105; single-peaked landscape 103f, 105
Flannery, T. 11–12, 46n5, 56, 57
Fligstein, N. 160n14, 169–70, 172
forum 'shopping' 86, 91n15
'forward-looking' attribution of responsibility 89
Foucault, M. 107n6
Fowler, J. 114
Fox, A. 86

Galbraith, J.K. 43–4
game-theoretic frameworks 90n6, 121n3
game theory 105, 107n3, 159n11
Gaventa, J. 102
Gavrilets, S. 107n7
General Linear Model (GLM) 50–1, 51f; limitations 51–2: (disproportional effects 54–5; interacting variables and separate effects 52–4)
generative mechanisms 22, 23–4, 27n8, 131–2, 134
Gerrits, L. 121n7
Giddens, A. 13, 118
Gilbert, N. 38, 66
Gladwell, M. 84, 153, 160n21, 171, 172, 173, 174, 178
goals 81, 90n9, 94
Goethe, J.W. von 71n4
Goldacre, Ben 127
Goldman Sachs 184–5n9
Goldthorpe, J. H.: on industrial relations 169; on political economy 99–100; on rational action 37–8, 71n7, 79–81, 82, 83, 89–90n4–5, 175; on social mobility 14, 20–1, 86–7, 91n16, 95, 101, 114, 117, 180
Goodwin, Fred 185n11
Gould, N. 122n12, 130
Gould, S.J. 40, 47n9, 56, 69, 107n8
Gramsci, A. 102
Granovetter, M. 18, 87, 98, 159n13
Great Society programmes 127–8, 140
green nudges 154–5

Gregg, P. 156
group-level selection 47m13

habits and conventions 35, 80, 82, 85, 86, 87, 150–1
habitual action 37–8, 79, 80, 83, 84, 88, 90n7, 110, 150
habitual world 90n11
habitus 91n12
Hacker, J.S. 181
Hager, N. 120, 160n15
Harford, T. 88
Harkness, S. 156
Harré, R. 22, 27n10, 41, 69, 78, 131
Hayek, F. 4, 19, 152
Haynes, L. et al. 129
Hayward, C.R. 89, 120, 183
Health Education England 119
Heath, A. et al. 84, 159n6
Hedström, P. 15, 16, 80
heuristics 80
hierarchical coordination 86
Hills, J. et al. 164
hinterland 98
Hirsch, F. 43, 94, 95–6, 97, 105–6, 107n1
Hirschman, A.O. 4, 20, 167
historical enquiry 89–90n4; see also Contingent Historical Model
Hobbes, T. 100
Hodgson, G.M. 31, 46n6
Hoggart, R. 120n1
Holland, J. 15, 18
House of Lords Science and Technology Committee 158n2
Howe, R.H. 71n4
human capital 165, 169
Hutton, W. 157

ideal types 24–5, 78, 159n10
'if-then' algorithms 35, 37, 47n11
imperative coordination 86–7, 88, 177
increasing returns 168
individualism 87, 105
inequality 106, 159n6, 164–5; addressing inequality 181–3; agile leaders on complex terrains 175–9; building positional advantage 170–5; under dynamic and disruptive change 166–8; rewards and their justification 168–70;
on stable and settled ground 165–6; understanding inequality 180–1
information 13, 18, 26n3, 35, 111, 176
innovation 66, 167, 184n7
insecurity 100, 106, 159n6
institutional analysis 26
institutional careers 173–4
institutional entrepreneurs 32–4, 39, 61, 159n10
institutional minimalism 86, 91n14
institutional venues 18
institutions 2, 18, 42; competing hopes 87; competing meanings and definitions of situation 87; competing memories 87; imperative coordination 86–7, 88, 177; rationale of 85–8
intellectual property rights 167, 176
international alliances 98

Jacobs, A. 70
Jacobs, Jane 114, 160n20
Jain, S. 64–6, 65f
Jervis, R. 51, 98, 121n3
John, P. et al. 157–8, 158n2, 158n5, 160n19
Jones, A. 91n15
Joseph, Sir Keith 89n3
Joyce, K.E. 143n7

Kahneman, D. 80, 111, 150
Kaldor, N. 13, 41, 71n8
Kant, I. 71n4
Kauffman, S.A. 3, 12, 107n7
Keynes, J.M. 4, 19, 43, 100, 105–6, 107n1, 150, 152, 167, 181, 182
Kingdon, J.W. 119
Klein, N. 120, 120–1n1, 122n14
Kleinwort Benson Bank 185n10
Koenig, M.D. et al. 66
Krishna, S. 64–6, 65f
Kristensen, P.H. 88, 153
Kuhn, T.S. 12–13, 52, 89n1, 160n16
Kupers, R. 194–5n1
Kuznets curve 164

Labour Government 127, 140, 149, 169
Langer, J. 53
Lauder, H. 107n2
Le Grand, J. 149

leadership 177; *see also* agile leaders on complex terrains
Leggett, W. 148, 158, 158n2, 158n5
leisure class 43, 160n18, 183
leverage 23, 40, 95
libertarian paternalism 147
Lieberson, S. 17, 20, 21, 24, 70, 99, 175
life chances 95–6
linear systems 50; *see also* General Linear Model
Loasby, B. 35, 38
local communities 153, 156
Lockwood, D. 91n16, 117
low peaks 39
Luke principle 181
Lukes, S.M. 78, 85, 89, 102, 107n5–6
Lundvall, B.-A. 167

McAdam, D. *et al.* 71n10
McAfee, A. 168
Malthus, T.R. 31–2, 46n3
marginal principle 184n4
marginal products 166
Marris, P. 27n9, 47n12
Marshall, T. H. 156
Marx, K. 13, 46n4, 167
material economy 43
Matthew principle 171, 181
Mau, S. 159n6
Mauss, M. 96
Maynard Smith, J. 60, 105
Mazzucato, M. 160n14, 167, 182
memes 32
mental models 18, 33, 39, 47n10, 87, 113, 116, 151, 159n10
meritocratic extremism 178
metis 90n10
Mill, J.S. 22
Millar, J. 149
misalignments 121n9, 121n10
models 78; and empirical data 24–5
moral claims 87
multi-level selection 47m13

national innovation systems 71n8, 167
natural selection 32, 33, 35, 38–9, 41–2, 46n3, 55
navigating complex environments 110–11; agile probing for positional advantage 112–14, 176; bounded rationality 111–12, 176; empirical investigation 116–18; policy applications 118–20; thresholds, alignments and sequences (TAS) 110, 114–16, 121–2n9–13; conclusion 120
Nelson, R.R. 118
neo-liberalism 158, 182
network analysis 97
Newton, I. 71n4
NICE (National Institute for Health and Clinical Excellence) 142n5
non-integral space 112
non-linearity 2, 10, 83; ideal types 24–5, 78, 159n10
normal science 52
North, D.C. 18, 85
nudge 118, 146–7, 148, 153, 158n5; action in the face of uncertainty 149–51
nuzzle 151–3, 158n5; policy nuzzles 153–5

Odling-Smee, F.J. *et al.* 32
Oliver, A. 148, 154, 157, 158n2, 158n5, 159n8
open systems 9, 53–4, 131
opportunism 171
'order for free' 12
organisational compliance 86
Ormerod, P. 19
Ostrom, E. 24, 86

Palier, B. 67
Papadopoulos, T. 98
Pareto, V. 180
path dependency 39; of evolution 38–9, 47n10, 55–6, 104; in policy 2, 37
Pawson, R. 22–3, 27n10, 129, 131–2, 137, 143n6–8
pecking order 96–7, 107n3, 121n9
Perri 6 18, 98
Pierson, P. 21, 54, 70n2, 99, 117, 159n12, 181
Piketty, T. 106, 164, 178
Polanyi, K. 4, 19, 182
Policy Horizons Canada 160n15
policy nuzzles 153–5
policy science and the evolutionary legacy 44–6
political economy 2, 99–100, 105, 183

politics 26
Pollan, M. 36
Popper, K.R. 77–9, 81–2, 83, 85, 89, 128
positional advantage 23, 42–3, 94–5; agile probing 112–14, 176; definition 94; and fitness landscapes 103–5, 103f, 113; implications for public policy 105–6; as occupation 100–1; one-dimensional view 95–7, 121n9; and power 95, 101–2; struggle for 34, 46n3; three-dimensional view 99–100, 106, 121n11; two-dimensional view 97–8, 121n10; *see also* first mover advantage; positional advantage creation
positional advantage creation 170–1; agile opportunism and 'luck' 171; beyond luck 174–5; closed doors and unexpected openings 171f, 172–3; and institutional careers 173–4
positional economy 43, 96
positional goods 96, 107n1
Potts, J. 13, 26n5, 39, 61, 99, 167
Powell, J.H. 62–4
power 23–4, 26, 27n9, 34, 47n12, 95, 101–2, 105, 170, 183
power laws 180
problem of control 41
problem of order 41
Protestant Ethic 78
public policy 1–2, 4–5, 19–20, 89; navigating complex environments 118–20; path dependency 2, 37; and positional advantage 105–6
'punctuated equilibria' 21, 24, 40, 54, 56
Puritan religious beliefs 90n8
purpose-rational (*zweckrational*) action 79, 80, 83, 90n5–6, 90n9

Qin Zhang 71n9
Qualitative Comparative Analysis (QCA) 71–2n10
qualitative system dynamics (QSD) 62–4, 63f
quantitative analysis of large-scale data sets (QAD) 81
quasi-experimental designs 128, 129

race for dynamic synergies 99, 103
racial discrimination 172, 175, 176, 183

racial segregation 15, 17, 20, 23, 24, 112, 114
Ragin, C.C. 71–2n10
randomised control trials (RCTs) 22, 127, 128–9, 129f, 142–3n5
rational action theory (RAT) 2, 17, 36, 37–8, 44, 46–7n7–8, 83; Goldthorpe on 37–8, 71n7, 79–81, 82, 83, 89–90n4–5, 175; varieties of 83–5
rational expectations theory 46n7, 111, 159n10
rationality principle 77–9, 81–2, 89
realism 22; evolutionary version 23, 134; ontological challenge 130–2, 132f, 143n6–7; *see also* transformative realism
Red Queen 105
reflection-in-action 177
reflective practitioners 130
reflexivity and routines 91n12
'rents' 100, 184n4
rewards *see* inequality
Rhodes, M.L. 121n7
Ricardo, D. 184n4
Ridge, T. 149
risk 150; *see also* uncertainty
Rogers, E. 167
Room, G. 16, 18, 21, 63, 102, 119, 180
Roumpakis, A. 98
rugged landscape 103f, 105
rules of thumb 37, 80, 84, 86, 89n2, 110, 150–1; in 'fast' thinking 112
runaway loops 62–3, 63f, 64

Sanderson, I. 143n7
Sayer, A. 164, 167
Scharpf, F.W. 86
Scheffer, M. *et al.* 67, 117
Schelling, T.C. 15, 16, 23, 24, 27n7, 80, 86, 112, 114, 183
Schön, D.A. 90n10, 177
Schumpeter, J.A. 32, 98, 167
Scott, J.C. 27n6, 90n10, 114, 143n6, 160n20
Secord, P. F. 78
self-organisation 3, 4, 9, 11; economic development 19–20; and the imposition of order 19–21; and positional advantage 104; social mobility 20–1

self-organised criticality 21, 24
selfish gene 32
sequences 115–16, 121–2n11–13
Sergot, M. 91n15
settled knowledge and practices 18, 79, 82, 84–5, 100, 173
shared prosperity 180
Simon, H.A. 18
single-peaked landscape 103f, 105
skill-biased 166
skills 165–6, 159
Skocpol, T. 71n10
Sloan Wilson, D. 47n13
'slow' thinking *see* 'fast' and 'slow' thinking
Smith, K.E. 143n7
social actors 85; agile probers and re-weavers of their world 84; as calculators of utility 83, 85, 91n13, 176; as followers of rules 83–4
social contracts 86, 106, 155, 156–7, 181
social emergence 12–14; macro-level 17–19; micro-actions and macro-changes 15–16; micro and macro in a linear world 14–15; transformative macro-dynamics 16–17
social experimentation 119
social investment state 156
social limits to growth 105
social mobility 14, 20–1, 86–7, 91n16, 95, 101, 114, 117, 180
social policy 45–6
social recession 159n6
social stratification 95, 171
societal 'problems' 70
sociological enquiry 89n4
sociology of control 9, 13, 16, 85, 86, 95
sociology of order 13, 17, 85, 86
Soros, G. 44
Squazzoni, F. 25
stable and settled ground 3, 165–6
Stackelberg games 107n3, 159n11
State education 149–50
statistical models 22
status group formation 178
Stewart, I. 26–7n6

Stewart, M. 113
Streek, W. 32
strong ties 87
structural balance 98
structural holes 97–8, 105, 112, 115
'struggle for existence' 11, 32, 34, 46n3, 55, 103
struggle to occupy the future 43, 100, 181
Sunstein, C.R. 80, 89n2, 112, 116, 146–8, 149, 150, 155, 158n4, 158n5
sustainability 106, 154–5
sustaining technologies 114
Sutcliffe, S. 130
Svalbard 10–11, 10f, 24

'tape of history' 56, 57, 69
Tavory, I. 90–1n11, 91n16
Tawney, R.H. 106, 155, 179
Teece, D.J. 184n7
templates 35–6
Thaler, R.H. 80, 89n2, 112, 116, 146–8, 149, 150, 155, 158n4, 158n5
Thatcher, Margaret 89n3, 169
Thelen, K. 32, 67
theory-building 22–4, 78
Thomas, J. L H. 107n4
threats and opportunities 87
thresholds 114–15, 121n9
Timmermans, S. 90–1n11, 91n16
tipping points 1–2, 15, 24, 40, 115, 117
Titmuss, R.M. 46
'tolerance schedule' 15
Tomaskovic-Devey, D. 169, 179
Toner, P. 41
transformative realism 3–4, 21–2, 23, 40, 69; in evidence-based policy-making 134–6, 135f; models and empirical data 24–5; race for dynamic synergies 99; theory-building 22–4; variables, actors and systems 25–6
Tree of Life 56, 56f, 57–8, 64, 65, 132, 133f
Troitzsch, K.G. 66
truth tables 72n10
Turner, R.H. 178

uncertainty 3, 17, 100, 111, 149–51, 159n10

value-rational (*wertrational*) action 79, 80, 87, 90n9
Veblen, T. 31, 36, 43, 44, 96, 106, 160n18, 183
venue 'shopping' 86, 91n15
Verplanken, B. 120n1
verstehende Soziologie 85
Von Bertalanffy, L. 69
Von Neumann, Richard 91n13

Wake, J. 185n10
Walras, M.-E.-L. 31, 36, 45
'war of each against all' 100
Watts, D. 114
weak signals 117
weak ties 87, 98, 159n13
wealth 100, 110, 120n1
wealth creation 167, 178, 181

wealth extraction 167, 178, 184–5n9
Weber, M. 13, 36–7, 71n4, 78, 79–80, 84, 85, 86, 90n8, 101, 110, 150, 178
'weightless' economy 87
wertrational (value-rational) action 79, 80, 87, 90n9
Weyman, A. *et al.* 148
'What Works' evidence centres for social policy 127
'wicked' problems 4
windfalls 168, 170, 178, 182, 184n7
winner-takes-all 99, 105–6, 164, 168, 171
Woolcock, M. 130
Wootton, B. 169
World Bank 180
Wright, S. 107n7

Zeitlin, J. 88, 153
zweckrational (purpose-rational) action 79, 80, 83, 90n5–6, 90n9